WORKING TOGETHER OR PULLING APART?

The National Health Service and child protection networks

Carol Lupton, Nancy North and Parves Khan

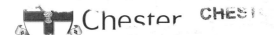Chester   CHES

The POLICY
P P
PRESS

First published in Great Britain in September 2001 by
The Policy Press
34 Tyndall's Park Road
Bristol BS8 1PY
UK

Tel +44 (0)117 954 6800
Fax +44 (0)117 973 7308
e-mail tpp@bristol.ac.uk
www.policypress.org.uk

British Library Cataloguing in Publication Data

A catalogue record for this book is available from the British Library

ISBN 1 86134 244 6

Carol Lupton is Reader in Applied Social Science and Director of the Social Services Research and Information Unit, University of Portsmouth. **Nancy North** is Principal Lecturer in Health Policy, University of Portsmouth. **Parves Khan** is Research Fellow, Department of Social Work, University of Southampton.

Cover design by Qube Design Associates, Bristol.

Printed and bound in Great Britain by Hobbs the Printers Ltd, Southampton.

Contents

Acknowledgements

We would like to express our thanks, first to Steve Hayes, from Portsmouth City Council for the original inspiration for the research underpinning much of this book and to the NHS Management Executive Research and Development Directorate (South West) for funding the empirical work. Also to Rose Storkey from Portsmouth City Council and Janet Feat from Hampshire County Council, for their help in crystallising the ideas contained herein and to Professor Sue Frost from the University of Huddersfield and Bruce Clark from the Department of Health for their helpful comments on individual chapters.

We also owe a considerable debt of gratitude to Darren Lacey, for collecting and analysing the data and to Debbie Adams and Jayne Sansom-Smith, from the Social Services Research and Information Unit (SSRIU) for essential secretarial assistance.

Last, but not least, we would like to thank all the professionals and managers in the three case study sites and from the Area Child Protection Committees (ACPCs) across the South East region who gave of their limited time to respond to our questions. We hope they feel that the end product fairly reflects their experiences and views. The final responsibility for the arguments and information contained in this book is, of course, our own.

Carol Lupton
Nancy North
Parves Khan

Introduction

These are not the opening paragraphs we would have wished to write. As we completed the final drafts of this book, news emerged of the abuse and eventual death of another young child. Anna Climbie was known to many of the local agencies responsible for child protection services: social services, the police and the health service. Understandably perhaps, the public again expressed disbelief at the apparent inability of these agencies to respond to the unmistakable signs of physical abuse endured by the little girl. Newspaper reports, and thus public debate, were quick to focus on the perceived failures of the professionals involved.

The response was also swift. The social services department (SSD) concerned was placed under 'special measures' and the social work case holder suspended pending an investigation into whether she and four other colleagues were to be disciplined. One of the police officers involved, although still at work, is reportedly facing a disciplinary inquiry and a total of eight officers are likely to be subject to internal investigation. Significantly, however, in the initial reaction to the event at least, relatively little public attention was paid to the role played by National Health Service (NHS) professionals. The actions of none of the health service's personnel who saw Anna in the months before her death, including, allegedly, a hospital paediatrician who considered her sores and marks to be self-inflicted, appear to have been subject to investigation by their agencies or professional associations. Although the formal inquiry has yet to be held, in the mind of the public and the press it is the performance of the social worker and, to an extent, the child protection police officers, that is widely seen to be the source of the problem.

As the 1989 Children Act and subsequent guidance make clear, however, effective child protection is a collective responsibility, involving the participation, to a greater or lesser extent, of a wide range of different agencies and professional groups. The NHS has a particularly important contribution to make to child protection, not least because of the number and diversity of its professional groups and services. Much research attention has been given to the problems of interagency collaboration involving the NHS (for example, Leathard, 1994; Soothill et al, 1995; Øvreteit et al, 1997), and some has examined interagency/professional collaboration in the specific context of child protection (for example, Stevenson, 1989; Blyth and Milner, 1990; Hallett, 1995; Birchall with

Hallett, 1995). Despite (or possibly because of) its diverse contribution, however, relatively little attention has been paid in the policy literature or in official child abuse inquiries to the specific role played by the NHS in child protection. This book is centrally about the role of the NHS and the contribution of its staff (both managers and professionals) to collaborative work at both central (policy development) and local (policy implementation) levels.

The in-depth focus of the book on the role of a particular agency provides its distinctive contribution to the child protection literature. It examines in detail the specific factors surrounding the organisation of the NHS that affect its potential for collaboration. Key chapters consider the performance of the health service in child protection, both historically and in the context of the Labour government's new modernisation agenda for the public sector. Chapter Five, for example, focuses on the internal 'power politics' of the NHS, exploring the changing nature of the relationship between different health professional groups, between professionals and NHS managers, and between the central and local levels of the service. The history of collaboration between health and social care service providers and the implications for 'partnership working' of new performance management and assessment frameworks are set out in Chapter Six. Description is then provided of the nature of, and issues surrounding, the child protection role of specific health professional groups such as the general practitioner (GP) (Chapter Nine), the health visitor (Chapter Ten) and the more recently established 'designated' and 'named' child protection professionals (Chapter Eight). Chapter Eleven provides an in-depth look at the experiences of health professionals working at the child protection 'front line' and highlights the key factors that appear to limit their ability (or inclination) to cooperate, either with other professional groups within the NHS or with professionals in other agencies.

The second distinctive characteristic of the book derives from its attempt to move beyond description of the difficulties surrounding interagency/ professional work to attempt an explanation of the reasons why collaboration has proved to be such an elusive policy ambition. The concern is to highlight the complex combination of factors that (potentially or actually) undermines attempts at joint working and affects the relationship between central policy development and its local implementation. In so doing, the text applies the theoretical insights of both the 'policy network' approach, developed most extensively in the UK by Marsh and Rhodes (Marsh and Rhodes, 1992; Rhodes, 1997;

Marsh, 1998) and the 'interorganisational analysis' of Benson in the US (Benson, 1975, 1983). After critically assessing the potential of these approaches for understanding the 'situated activity' of child protection (Chapter One), the text sets out the key characteristics of the national and local networks in the child protection policy arena (Chapter Two). This chapter also details the role of central regulation and guidance in establishing the 'mandated coordination' of the child protection system for England and Wales. Chapter Seven examines the key role played by the Area Child Protection Committees (ACPCs) as a central layer – a 'system within a system' (Sanders, 1999) – between the prescriptions of the central policy community and their implementation (or not) by local delivery or 'provider networks'.

The text is also distinctive in its concern with the 'dynamics' as well as the structures of interprofessional/multiagency cooperation. The theoretical frameworks employed, particularly that of Benson's interorganisational analysis, enable a focus on the relationships within the network as well as on the network in its wider social and political environment. This illuminates the susceptibility of interprofessional/ agency collaboration to external changes such as public sector reorganisation, for example, or shifts in service or disciplinary paradigms. It also helps us understand the ways in which the operation of networks is underpinned by the need for participating agencies to maximise their 'market positions' and by the impact of social relations of power and influence that characterise the wider policy sector, and society, more generally. Particular attention is paid to the role of 'knowledge' within child protection networks and to the impact of 'disciplinary dynamics' (professional power struggles) on interprofessional collaboration (Chapter Three). Chapter Four examines the impact on collaboration of variations in the forms of governance, accountability and regulation surrounding the different agencies and professional groups working within the child protection network. It considers whether the creation of the mixed economy of welfare has served to make collaboration more difficult by increasing the diversity of organisational players and making more complex the issues of regulation and accountability.

In developing this agenda, the text draws heavily, although not exclusively, on the findings of a large-scale empirical investigation of the role of health professionals in child protection undertaken by the authors between 1996 and 1999. Funded by the NHS Executive (South and West), this study aimed to describe the role then played by a range of health groups (professionals and managers) within child protection and to identify, from the perspectives of those groups and their counterparts outside the NHS, the factors which appeared to facilitate or impair their contribution to local child protection networks. It was anticipated that these factors would operate at the interpersonal, interprofessional and interorganisational levels as well as being subject to wider developments at the 'supra-organisational' level. In contrast to the fairly extensive attention given in the literature to the impact of interpersonal and interprofessional factors, relatively little attention has been paid to the effect of changes within and between the organisations involved or to the impact on those organisations of wider social and political developments.

The study involved a 'nested' mixed method design, combining a series of in-depth case studies in three health authority areas with a regional postal survey of all members of the ACPCs across the South West region (n=140, 60% response rate). The case study investigations involved self-completion questionnaires to all 'front-line' professionals attending child protection conferences over the six months prior to the fieldwork (n=175, 47% response rate); non-participant observation of those conferences (n=120); researcher interviews with 'strategic' level personnel in all agencies represented on the ACPCs (n=67, 100% response rate), with the 'designated' and 'named' child protection professionals (n=19, 90% response rate) and with GPs in two of the health authority areas (n=100, response rates of 21% and 60%). The collection of primary data was accompanied by a literature review and analysis of secondary data sources. Discussion of the research and its findings can be found in a range of academic and professional publications (Lupton and Khan, 1998; Lupton et al, 1999a, 2000; Khan et al, 1999a, 1999b; North et al, 1999, 2000) as well as in the final report of the study (Lupton et al, 1999b).

This book, however, is not just about the NHS and its role in child protection; it is also about the policy process more widely and, in particular, about the relationship between policy making and policy implementation or 'outcome'. Ever since the establishment of the British welfare state, effective collaboration between its constituent sectors, agencies and provider groups has remained an enduring policy problem, apparently unresponsive to the plethora of central initiatives devised for its resolution. The greater fragmentation of the state that occurred during the 1980s and 1990s, with the emergence of a range of intermediary agencies and the development of public sector markets, has arguably increased the potential gap between central policy objectives and their local implementation. This process of 'hollowing out' the state has made the business of governing more difficult as the role of the central state is increasingly reduced to that of 'steering' rather than 'rowing' (Osborne and Gaebler, 1992, p 45) the activities of its diverse advisory bodies, executive agencies and regional outposts.

At the same time as the coordinating capacity of the state has lessened, however, there has been a growing political recognition that some of the more enduring or 'wicked' (6, P., 1997) social problems facing modern society require more integrated or 'cross-cutting' policy solutions. The ability to implement such solutions, however, will depend as crucially on the effectiveness of local collaborative arrangements as it will on the quality or quantity of central policy directives or 'mandates'. The focus of this text is on the (external and internal) factors that encourage or undermine multiagency and interprofessional collaboration in the specific policy context of child protection. As such, it is hoped that its discussions will advance understanding of the ways in which that such collaboration can be improved. In so far as its analysis identifies factors that are generalisable across policy sectors or to other areas of 'situated activity', however, it is also hoped that this book will have relevance wider than the child protection context.

ONE

Models and metaphors: the theoretical framework

Introduction

The idea of policy networks assumed growing importance in the public policy literature of the 1990s. Defined as "(more or less) stable patterns of social relations between interdependent actors, which take shape around policy problems and/or policy programmes" (Kikert et al, 1997, p 6), the concept emerged originally in the US in the early 1950s as a critique of pluralistic explanations of political decision making. Pluralist theory posits a (more or less unlimited) number of groups competing (with more or less equal degrees of influence) for the attention of a largely disinterested state. Network analysis in contrast argues that a small number of groups enjoy a privileged relationship with the state at the expense of other interests. The approach was given particular form in the concept of 'iron triangles': a metaphor for the symbiotic relationship seen to exist between policy makers, government agencies and selected interest group(s) within a particular area of policy making (Peters, 1986).

As well as being distinct from pluralist analysis, network theory also differed from the other main model of interest group representation: corporatism. Unlike pluralism, in which all pressure groups are seen to have a roughly equal ability to influence the policy process, corporatist theory highlights the privileged role of certain, selected groups. Because of their key role in society, these groups have a 'representational monopoly' (Schmitter, 1979) that is recognised, licensed or created by the state. In the UK, for example, corporatism described the relationship between the state and the organised representatives of 'capital' and 'labour' that characterised the development of economic and industrial policy in the 1960s and early 1970s (Cawson, 1986). Despite obvious similarities to their own approach, policy network theorists such as Marsh and Rhodes (Marsh and Rhodes, 1992; Rhodes, 1997; Marsh, 1998) argue that the corporatist model may only be applicable in certain contexts. Policy making is more complex than the corporatists suggest. Rather than taking a 'monolithic' view of policy making, which sees all areas of government policy dominated by the same powerful groups, Marsh and Rhodes argue that it is important to "disaggregate policy analysis" (Marsh and Rhodes, 1992, p 4) and examine the particular forms of interest group representation that characterise specific policy areas. Although it is likely that policy making will always be characterised by the involvement of a fairly restricted number of groups, the precise nature of these groups, they suggest, will vary between policy areas.

As with both pluralist and corporatist approaches, the focus of policy network analysis is on policy development at a national level. The achievement of central policy ambitions such as better interagency collaboration, however, will depend crucially on the relationship between central policy networks and those responsible for policy implementation at the local level. To understand the nature of local service delivery or 'provider networks' and their relationship to policy-making networks, this chapter draws on the 'interorganisational network' approach developed by Benson in the US (1975, 1983). This approach understands a particular policy sector as a mini 'political economy' in which there may be many networks operating on a number of different, interrelated levels. The focus of interorganisational analysis is on the internal and external dynamics of these networks. Its concern is to understand the relationships within and among networks and between those networks and the policy sector, and society, more widely. In addition to illuminating policy making at central government level, therefore, interorganisational analysis may be helpful in understanding the policy implementation or 'delivery' networks and the nature of the relationship between the two. Before examining these models and assessing how well they apply to the child protection context, the chapter briefly identifies some of the key changes in public administration that took place during the 1980s and 1990s which provide the wider context for the development of child protection policy and, some argue, for the increased centrality of policy networks to the organisation of the central state.

The political context

As we have indicated, the idea of policy networks has to be understood in the context of the major changes in the role of the state that took place in most Western economies over the latter years of the 20th century. A combination of factors, including economic depression and an ideological distrust of 'big government' led to growing public disenchantment with the performance (and cost) of the social democratic state (Wright, 1994; Hood, 1995; Rhodes, 1997). This prompted what some have termed a 'reinvention of government' (Osborne and Gaebler, 1992) in which the traditional bureaucratic way of running the state gave way to a new approach to public sector management. Most commentators agree that this 'new public management' (NPM) involves the combination of at least two central strands: a new 'institutional economics' (fostering competition and choice) and a professionalisation of managerial expertise (ensuring the 'freedom to manage') (Pollitt, 1990). Cutler and Waine (1994) argue that UK public sector development has been characterised by what they call the 'corporate capitalist' variant of NPM. This is seen to comprise three key elements: tighter political control over public expenditure, decentralisation of managerial responsibility and the development of new managerialist principles (target setting, performance measurement, performance-related pay, and so on). In the UK at least (although not universally; see Walsh, 1995) these three strands were accompanied by a politically inspired drive towards privatisation.

The growth of NPM resulted in significant changes in the organisation and delivery of public sector services. The separation of policy making from the administration of services, the blurring of the boundaries between public and private organisations and the increased dominance of market mechanisms (such as contracts and competitive tendering) resulted in more fragmented and diverse service structures. A large number of agencies sprang up which operated somewhere between the central and the local state and between public and private spheres. These 'intermediate bodies' comprised a range of different types of organisations with a variety of functions, including executive 'Next Steps' agencies, regional executives, 'quangos' and private/not-for-profit providers. Their key characteristics were their 'distance' from central government departments and their relative autonomy or 'freedom to manage' (Marr, 1995). As the state no longer directly delivered services but transferred them to a variety of intermediate bodies, its role increasingly became one of 'steering' not 'rowing' (Osborne and Gaebler, 1992) the operation of the public sector. In turn, commentators have argued, this 'hollowing out' or fragmentation of the state requires a shift from the notion of government to the idea of governance. Broader than government, governance is the means by which the interrelations between society, the market and the increasingly fragmented central state are ordered:"Governance reflects a 'differentiated polity' ... characterised by functional and institutional specialisation and the fragmentation of policies and politics" (Rhodes, 1997, p 7).

There is disagreement about the extent to which the breaking up or 'hollowing out' of the state has strengthened or weakened central political control. Some, such as Saward (1997), argue that it has enabled more effective control, by separating the making of policies (politics) from their operationalisation (administration). Combined with stronger central regulation, this separation has given governments the best of both worlds. Governing at 'arm's-length' enables politicians to distance themselves, when necessary, from the responsibility for policy development while at the same time increasing political scrutiny and control over its implementation. In particular, many suggest that hollowing out has improved the ability of the central state to control both professionals and bureaucrats. Subject to the disciplines of NPM rather than the ethos of public service, it is argued that the new professional manager is less resistant to political control than the traditional bureaucrat (Massey, 1993). Those providing services are increasingly constrained by the disciplines of the market as well as by tighter inspection and regulation systems. In addition, new managerialist mechanisms such as career restructuring, performance-related pay and management by contract may make professional activity more transparent, thus heightening its susceptibility to increased managerial (and political) control (Stewart and Walsh, 1992).

Others, however, question how far these changes have actually strengthened central political control. Many identify a persistent gap between policy intent and policy implementation and question how effectively central government is able to regulate or 'steer' semi-autonomous delivery agencies. In this view, the 'implementation gap' is made worse by the fragmentation of the state, which hampers the development of a coordinated and coherent policy response. The result, it is argued, is that the government is less able to confront intractable or 'wicked' (6, P., 1997) social problems, such as exclusion, unemployment or child abuse, which require 'cross-cutting' policy solutions. On the international scene, the new millennium brought signs of growing concern about the extent to which the precepts of NPM have diminished, rather than increased, the effectiveness of the state. The acknowledgement of a certain tension between 'new managerialism' and 'good governance' reflects a broader shift of policy focus from the early neo-Liberal concern to minimalise the state to growing interest in ways of making its operation more effective (World Development Report, 1997).

Policy-making networks

Networks, as we have indicated, are seen as particularly appropriate to the analysis of policy making within the 'differentiated polity' of the hollowed out state. There is considerable debate, however, about what networks are and how they operate. For a start there is disagreement about whether networks actually exist. Some argue that the idea of networks should be viewed as an abstract model, or 'metaphor' (Dowding, 1994; Peters, 1986); an analytical perspective, like pluralism or corporatism, designed to help us understand interest group politics. Others insist that networks are a new, empirically real, form of political governance: "... a real change in the structure of the polity" (Mayntz, 1994, p 5). Related to this, and reflecting the enduring structure/agency debate in political thought more widely, network theorists also differ on the question of whether networks are to be understood as structural relationships between political institutions (Marsh and Rhodes, 1992; Klijn, 1997) or as interpersonal relationships between key actors (Richardson and Jordan, 1979; Wilkes and Wright, 1987; Dowding, 1995).

There is further disagreement about the level at which networks operate. Some argue (Smith, 1993) that they are relevant to the development of policy across a whole area or sector of central state practice (for example, health policy); others contend that they may be more important, or equally important, in understanding policy generation at sub-sectoral level (for example, acute care, primary health care, social care) (Jordan et al, 1994). There are also differences of opinion about whether the analysis of network activity should focus at the 'macro level' of central state activity (theories about the nature of the state), at the 'meso level' (the dynamics of pressure/interest group politics) or at the 'micro level' of individual behaviour and rational choice. Finally, there is also lack of unanimity about the extent to which and ways in which the operation of networks affects policy outcomes. Some, such as Daugbjerg and Marsh (1998) suggest they have a determining influence; others, such as Hay (1998), suggest that networks may have a partial affect; yet others, such as Dowding (1995), argue that networks in and of themselves (as opposed to the behaviour of those within them) have no influence on policy making.

The most developed assessment of policy network theory in the UK is provided in the work of Marsh and Rhodes (Rhodes, 1981; Marsh and Rhodes, 1992; Marsh, 1998). This effectively offers a compromise on most of the above dilemmas. On the question of structure versus agency, for example, these authors argue the importance of understanding networks as "structures of resource dependency" (Marsh, 1998, p 11). At the same time, however, Marsh (1998) concedes that network analysis must also recognise the fact that the behaviour of its composite members (their rational choices) will affect the operation of the network. What is needed, he argues, is recognition of the 'dialectical nature' of the relationship between network structure and individual behaviour: "We need to recognise that, while networks shape preferences, the actions of agents mediate and renegotiate these structural constraints" (1998, p 70).

In the same way, Marsh and Rhodes also argue that policy networks can be seen to operate at either or both the sectoral and sub-sectoral level. Which level is more important will depend on the particular policy area being studied and the relationship between the different levels may be of particular relevance. Further, although policy networks are located at the 'meso level', Marsh and Rhodes suggest that analysis must also take account of the fact that their operation is affected by external processes that impact on both their structure and composition. These wider 'exogenous' forces have to be explained with reference to theories about the nature of the state ('macro level') and its articulation with civil society as well as by 'micro level' examination of the behaviour of network members as "... strategically calculating agents" (Marsh, 1998, p 195). Currently, however, these authors concede, the relationship between these different levels of analysis – sectoral and sub-sectoral and macro, meso and micro – is underdeveloped in the policy network literature.

Developing Heclo's (1978) theory of the move from 'iron triangles' to 'issue networks' as the dominant form of policy making, Marsh and Rhodes establish a continuum of policy network types. These range from tight-knit policy communities at the one end (few participants and a balance of power) which share basic values, exchange resources and engage in frequent and high-quality interaction based on consensus, to the looser-limbed issue networks at the other (many participants of unequal power) characterised by fluctuating interaction with limited, or no consensus. Unlike Heclo, however, Marsh and Rhodes do not assume that a general shift has occurred within the modern state from the dominance of policy communities to that of issue networks. Empirical applications of their typology in policy sectors such as agriculture (Smith, 1993), sea defences (Cunningham, 1992), health (Wistow, 1992) and nuclear power (Saward, 1993), they argue, indicate that different policy sectors are characterised by different types of network, although all involve limited access to the policy process. Policy dominance by issue networks, however, they suggest, is likely to be rare, occurring only where there are no powerful economic, producer or professional groups with vested interests. Typically such networks operate at the margins of the policy agenda (Marsh and Rhodes, 1992, p 254).

Haywood and Hunter's (1982) study of 'older persons' policy formation in the NHS of the early 1980s would seem to reinforce this conclusion. Although a wider 'issue community' was found to exist, they argue that it remained dominated by an 'iron core' of central departmental officials, medical professionals and two 'producer groups' – the Royal College of Nursing and the British Geriatric Society. The involvement of a greater number of groups in the consultation process, they warn, should not in itself be taken to signify a lessening of control by a closed inner core: "... iron triangles may be less exclusive because some policies are processed in an extended range of groups [but] a closed system can still operate" (1982, p 161). Jordan (1981) argues, however, that it may not be appropriate to view iron triangles and issue networks as "... discretely different arrangements" (1981, p 103); it is possible for an issue network to display characteristics of an iron triangle, but with "... a greatly increased population, with a further disaggregation of power, with less predictable participants [and] with reduced cohesion and homogeneity" (p 103).

Other empirical applications of the network approach go further still and suggest that it may be possible for a particular policy sector or sub-sector to be characterised by more than one type of network. Thus Read's study (1992) of smoking policy revealed a core community (ministers and officials at the then Department of Health and Social Security, and the tobacco companies) surrounded by a wider issue network comprising groups such as the British Medical Association (BMA) and the Action on Smoking and Health (ASH). A similar differentiation of 'core' and 'peripheral' policy networks was also found in the analysis of the agricultural (Smith, 1993), nuclear power (Saward, 1992) and youth unemployment (Marsh, 1992) policy communities. Marsh and Rhodes resist this extension of their framework, insisting that such distinctions only serve to obscure the boundaries of networks. That these boundaries are permeable, they contend, should not detract from the qualitative difference between those responsible for developing policy and any other interested parties who may subsequently be consulted on that policy or attempt to influence its development. The key characteristic of an issue network, as opposed to that of other interested or 'attentive parties', they argue, is that the former, although larger and less cohesive, nevertheless retains the central characteristics of a network, involving: "... stable, regulated and predictable relations" (Jordan, 1981, p 121).

Limitations of the policy network approach

Useful though the idea of the policy network is for identifying the key groups and interests involved in a particular area of policy development, the approach has some important limitations for our focus on interagency collaboration in child protection. These are of two basic kinds, but both stem from the relative lack of attention paid by policy network theorists to the dynamics of networks. Despite acknowledging the relevance of the relationships within and between networks, and between networks and their wider environment, relatively little attention is paid to these dimensions. The attempt to construct a typology of network forms moreover almost inevitably results in a tendency to emphasise structure at the expense of process. In particular, the stress on the existence of consensus between network participants may have led network theorists to underplay the internal conflicts and tensions within networks and their impact on the subsequent development of policy (Peters, 1986). As a result, Hay argues, policy network theory has produced an overly static theoretical framework that fails to acknowledge the extent to which networks operate as sites of contested or 'strategic action' (Hay, 1998, p 35). Marsh and others acknowledge this problem and the need for a "more dynamic, dialectical approach" (1998, p 196) which would examine the influence of exogenous factors, not just on the structure and composition of the network but also on the shifting interests, power and resources of the actors within it.

The second relative limitation of the policy network framework derives from its uni-dimensional focus. Although it is acknowledged that networks may operate at the sub-sectoral (for example, social care, youth justice, farming, chemicals) as well as sectoral (for example, health, policing, agriculture, industry) level, the nature of the relationship has not been given much attention in the literature. As Marsh and Rhodes concede: "The articulation between sectoral and sub-sectoral levels needs further analysis" (1992, p 255). Arguably, moreover, in many areas of policy activity, the basic two-fold model of sectoral and sub-sectoral is likely to prove too restrictive. As Ham (1999) suggests in the context of the NHS, the national policy network (he prefers the term 'community') is fragmented into a series of sub-communities organised around key issues such as older people, abortion, substance misuse and so on. The interactions between these sub-communities and relevant sectoral level networks may be crucial to understanding specific areas of policy development. Just as crucial, indeed, may be the relationship between different policy networks, at either sectoral or sub-sectoral level. Thus Smith's (1993) analysis of the government's policy on eggs reveals the importance of the sectoral-level clash between the health and agriculture policy networks. Finally, and most importantly, the relationship between policy development networks and service delivery or 'provider networks' will be central to our understanding of the factors affecting the gap between central policy objectives and their implementation at a local level. Again, however, this relationship has been paid little detailed attention within the policy network literature.

Interorganisational networks

One approach that may be more useful in examining the internal and contextual dynamics of policy networks is the 'interorganisational analysis' developed by Benson in the US (1975, 1983). For Benson, specific policy sectors (such as health, employment) are seen as complex interorganisational phenomena, involving many different networks and operating on a number of different levels. Networks are defined fairly broadly as "… a number of distinguishable organisations having a significant amount of interaction with one another" (1975, p 230). Within networks participants are connected to each other by a series of mutual resource dependencies and their relationships may be direct or indirect, consensual or competitive: "Such interaction may at one extreme include extensive, reciprocal changes of resources or intense hostility and conflict at the other" (p 230). The problem with much analysis, Benson argues, is that it has tended to theorise the operation of these networks, and the wider policy sector itself, as somehow 'context free'. In contrast, he argues, it is important to understand that their operation is embedded in, and subject to the operation of, wider political and economic processes.

For Benson, then, analysis of the operation of interorganisational networks must focus on two different 'sets' of concepts. The first 'set', which has characterised much traditional policy analysis, centres on the patterns of interaction that derive from organisations' collaboration in the performance of their core functions. For Benson this interaction can be understood in terms of the achievement of equilibrium across four key dimensions: domain consensus (agreement regarding the appropriate role and scope of each agency); ideological consensus (agreement regarding the nature of the tasks faced and the most appropriate way of approaching these tasks); positive evaluation (by workers in one organisation of the work of those in others); and work coordination (alignment of working patterns and culture). Those networks in strong equilibrium are characterised by highly coordinated, cooperative interactions, based on consensus and mutual respect.

Applying a basic systems theory approach, Benson's broad hypothesis is that these components of equilibrium are related, so that improvements (or decline) on one dimension will bring improvements (or decline) in others. Significant areas of imbalance are possible, however, and will affect the operation of the network. Thus a network may be characterised by a high degree of ideological and domain consensus and mutually positive evaluation of each other's roles but experience a poor level of work coordination. Equally there may be agreement about the role of the respective agencies and a high degree of work coordination, but little positive evaluation of each agency's contribution. Yet again, networks may display high levels of work coordination as a result of central policy prescription (mandated cooperation), but experience working relationships based on mutual distrust or limited understanding of each other's roles and ways of working. As a result, individual networks may be subject to one of three different types of operational imbalance: forced coordination (high on work coordination, low on domain and ideological consensus and mutual evaluation); consensual inefficiency (high on all other attributes, but low levels of work coordination); or evaluative imbalance (high on work cooperation and strong domain and ideological consensus, but low on positive evaluation).

To understand why a particular organisational network has the 'surface' characteristics it does, Benson argues that it is necessary to examine a second set of concepts. These relate to factors that operate beneath the surface (superstructure) at the 'substructural' level. Although having some degree of autonomy, interactions on the cultural or 'superstructural' level are underpinned by "deeper and more fundamental processes" (1975, p 231) which influence the behaviour of participating organisations. These underlying factors relate to the participants' own organisational objectives: the fulfilment of programme requirements (key service delivery objectives); the maintenance of a clear domain of high social importance (ensuring or enhancing public legitimacy and support for the service agenda); the maintenance of orderly, reliable patterns of resource flow (ensuring adequate funding); and the application and defence of the organisation's paradigm (the 'technological–ideological commitment' to certain ways of working) (see Figure 1). As a result, the dynamics of an interorganisational network should be viewed as a mini 'political economy' in which the behaviour of each participant is determined in large part by its need to secure these

Figure 1: The 'political economy' of an interorganisational network

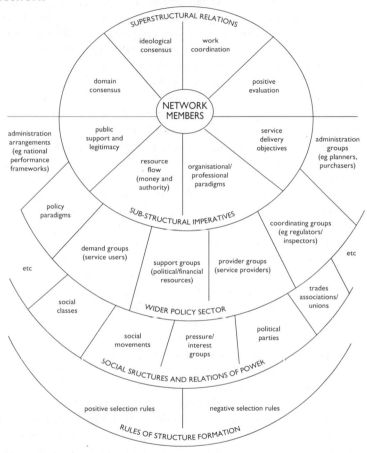

SUPERSTRUCTURAL RELATIONS

ideological consensus

work coordination

domain consensus

positive evaluation

NETWORK MEMBERS

administration arrangements (eg national performance frameworks)

public support and legitimacy

service delivery objectives

administration groups (eg planners, purchasers)

resource flow (money and authority)

organisational/ professional paradigms

policy paradigms

SUB-STRUCTURAL IMPERATIVES

coordinating groups (eg regulators/ inspectors)

etc

demand groups (service users)

support groups (political/financial resources)

provider groups (service providers)

etc

social classes

WIDER POLICY SECTOR

trades associations/ unions

social movements

pressure/ interest groups

political parties

SOCIAL SRUCTURES AND RELATIONS OF POWER

positive selection rules

negative selection rules

RULES OF STRUCTURE FORMATION

Acknowledgements (and apologies) to Benson (1975, 1983)

'external' objectives. Achievement of domain or ideological consensus within the network, effective work cooperation or positive mutual evaluation will be possible only to the extent that it does not involve actions that undermine the market position of the collaborating agency. As Benson argues: "Agencies can agree on matters of domain and ideology only to the extent that such agreement does not threaten their interests" (1975, p 237).

However, it is also clear that not all organisations collaborating within an interorganisational network will possess the same degree of power, resources or legitimacy. Some participants therefore may be in a better position to defend and enhance their wider organisational objectives than others. The relative power of organisations within the network derives from two main sources. First, from their role within the network whereby certain organisations have a more central function than others (for example, those like child protection sections of SSDs which are at the centre of the 'referral flow' or those, such as health, that may be seen to have access to a wide range of relevant services). Second, network power will derive from the organisation's linkages to wider patterns of social organisation (parties/classes/social movements/interest groups and so on). Thus the role of the NHS in interagency networks, for example, is likely to be enhanced by the strong professional power of its provider groups. The organisational weight of criminal justice agencies, in contrast, will derive from the strength of political and public support for the law and order agenda. Yet others, such as social services, may derive power from the sheer number of user/interest groups which have a stake in their services. Ideology, defined as the way of talking about, and seeking legitimacy for, an agency's own 'technology' (sphere of organisational expertise) is also important in affecting the flow of resources to network participants. In many cases, Benson argues, ideological claims may stand in place of claims to technical expertise and it may in practice often be difficult, particularly in human services agencies, to differentiate the two: "... the line between ideology and technology is often hazy because treatment often consists of the transmission of attitudes and values" (1975, p 237).

This relative power of collaborating organisations within a network can be used in a variety of ways, including the ability to 'reach across' into weaker agencies and determine their policies and practices, or to determine the pattern of the resource flow within or between networks. It may be used to block the claims of agencies with different or competitive organisational paradigms or to control or even 'licence' the service activities of weaker agencies. Thus the relative power of medical professionals may be seen to have colonised many areas of health and social care provision and constrained the role and authority of other professionals, such as nurses or social workers (see Chapter Five). Some networks may not be characterised by easily identifiable power imbalances, but may comprise a broad balance of power between the different participants. In such situations, Benson argues, the operation of the network may experience difficulty: "Such networks are often blocked and non-co-operative because

... none can muster power sufficient to dictate terms to the others" (1975, p 235).

In Benson's analysis, however, the operation of an interorganisational network must be understood in its wider context (a political economy within a political economy). This context provides the basic 'terms and conditions' under which the network operates, affecting crucially both the supply of resources (money and authority) to a network, its structure and the relationships within it. The particular context of each network will vary, although different networks may experience overlapping environments. This context moreover will exist on many levels. On the first, most immediate, level it will comprise the administrative arrangements (for example, balance of public/private provision, lines of political and managerial accountability) and service paradigms (for example, social versus medial model) that characterise the wider policy sector. Tensions may arise when the network's operation cuts across other policy sectors characterised by different service structures or operational paradigms. Changes in these wider paradigms or administrative structures will have direct implications for the operation of networks by altering the mix of resource dependencies within them. Indeed, as Benson (1983) points out, service reorganisation may be deliberately designed to alter the patterns of resource dependencies underpinning interorganisational networks, especially at front-line levels. Thus, for example, the explicit intention of the UK public sector reform during the 1980s and 1990s was to increase the role of private and independent sector providers, relative to that of state.

In turn, the wider environment of the network is itself affected by the operation of a 'deeper set of rules'. These derive from two sources: from power and interest group structures and from the rules of 'structure formation'. The operation of any policy sector (and its constituent networks) will be influenced by the particular combination of 'structured interests' (Alford, 1975) embedded within it. These interests may involve a combination of any of the following: demand groups (service users); support groups (those providing political or financial resources); administrative groups (agency administrators/planning agencies); provider groups (those delivering services); and coordinating groups (those charged with regulation, inspection and the processes of 'good governance'). The dynamic of a particular policy sector derives from the tensions within and between these different interest groups as well as from changes in wider administrative arrangements and policy paradigms. Generally, the operation of a particular sector will tend to enhance the interests of some groups at the expense of others. It will also resist any change in administrative arrangements or policy paradigms that may threaten these established interests. In turn, the power-interest structure of any policy area is likely to be explicable in respect of the power relations that characterise society more widely. In this way, for example, Gough (1979) and others link the emergence of the welfare state to the post-war 'settlement' between the interest of 'capital' and 'labour'.

Ultimately, for Benson, in the last analysis the operation of a particular policy sector is constrained by the fundamental rules of 'structure formation', deriving from the nature and operation of the state in advanced capitalist societies. These rules are of two kinds: negative selection rules (those that would violate the essential character of the capitalist state) and positive selection rules (those that contribute to the effective reproduction of the social formation). These rules restrict the policy sector's room to manoeuvre but are not immutable: "Negotiations and bargains occur within the range of available alternatives" (1983, p 160). They do, however, place ultimate boundaries on the operation of the sector which cannot be crossed without "eliciting a counteraction" (p 161). They may also, from time to time, occasion significant structural reorganisation within that sector as emerging contradictions undermine established relations. In this way the ongoing process of reorganisation in the health and social care policy sectors has been linked to the inherent crises of capital accumulation which restricts the welfare capacity of the state (Offe, 1975). Analysis of the relationships within and between interorganisational networks, Benson argues, must take account of the existence of these deeper 'macro structural' rules; there is more to networks than resource-driven exchanges or 'games': "By taking a broader view over a longer-term, we can see that the games form patterns; that the exchanges operate with institutionally governed resources; that the games are connected, with some taking priority over others; that there are some limits or boundaries within which the games are played" (1983, p 164).

Conclusion

As we have argued, the 'policy network' approach offers an important starting point for the analysis of the specific policy area of child protection. Its typology of network characteristics provides a useful means to identify the structure of the child protection policy community and the particular combinations of interests involved in (and those excluded from) the policy-making process. A basic question for our analysis of child protection is, therefore, the extent to which the policy area is characterised by the close-knit, restricted combination of interests seen to typify the 'policy community' end of the continuum or involves the operation of a more diffuse and inclusive 'issue network'. Despite the resistance of Marsh and Rhodes to the idea of a combination of network types, moreover, existing empirical applications of network theory suggest the possibility of a combination of 'core' and 'peripheral' networks that may be of relevance to a complex, multi-level policy area such as child protection.

The value of the policy network approach, however, as an explanatory theoretical framework, is limited by its relative inattention to the dynamics of networks. There is little in the basic framework that can help us understand the factors influencing the internal relationships of networks or the operation of networks in their wider context. This is not helped by the restricted focus of policy network theorists on policy development at governmental (or sub-governmental) level. Almost no attention is paid to the nature and operation of those networks involved in policy implementation or delivery. Yet the nature of these policy delivery networks, and their relationship to policy making, is central to our understanding of the child protection system. It is also central to the analysis of the 'implementation gap'; the enduring space between policy ambition and policy outcome.

In respect of these aspects of the policy process, Benson's more fluid and dynamic model provides a complementary approach. In particular, the four key dimensions of equilibrium – 'domain consensus', 'ideological consensus', 'positive evaluation' and 'work coordination' – offer a helpful framework for the analysis of the internal dynamics of the multiagency and interprofessional networks operating in child protection. Benson's approach can assist our understanding of the impact of external factors on the internal dynamics of a network. These derive from the basic organisational imperatives constraining the actions of network participants, the administrative structures and policy paradigms of the wider policy sector and the structured interests embedded within society more generally.

In combination, therefore, the two approaches would seem to have something to offer as a broad overall theoretical framework for the investigation of the child protection policy process. The typologies of network analysis may help to reveal the characteristics of the policy development network at central government level and Benson's interorganisational analysis may serve to illuminate the operation of more peripheral issue networks and/or those involved in multiagency service delivery networks at a local level. The latter may also help us understand the nature of the links between the two types of network and thus the factors influencing the relationship between policy development and implementation. Despite the insights of these two approaches, however, much remains to be determined by detailed empirical analysis, including the precise configuration of the network(s) involved in any selected policy context, the particular balance of power and interest within them and the nature of their relationship with the other networks, organisational structures and policy paradigms that make up the wider policy arena. The next chapter begins this process by examining the nature of the networks that comprise the child protection 'policy architecture' for England and Wales.

TWO

Policy communities and provider networks in child protection

Introduction

As identified in Chapter One, 'policy networks' are seen to play a key role in the policy-making process. The idea of networks, we have argued, may be particularly appropriate in a multiagency, interprofessional area such as child protection. The limitations of network theory for the analysis of child protection policy, however, have also been outlined. In particular, we suggested that the operation of networks in their wider contexts, their interaction with other networks and the relationship between policy-making and policy-delivery networks have been relatively neglected within the relevant literature. These limitations may be especially problematic in the field of child protection where, as we shall indicate below, the networks are highly susceptible to external pressures and are cross-sectoral and multilevel in nature. Moreover, although the possibility of internal conflict is theorised in certain types of network (those closer to the 'issue network' than to the 'policy community' end of the continuum), little attention has been paid to this dimension and its impact on policy outcomes. Again, we would suggest, the analysis of internal tension or conflict rather than cohesion and consensus may be particularly relevant to the politically sensitive area of child protection.

A complementary framework for understanding the operation of policy networks, we argue, is that developed by Benson (1975, 1983). This sees the policy arena as an interorganisational 'political economy' comprising many different networks. Collaboration (within or between networks) is characterised by tensions deriving from the unequal resources and authority of network members, underpinned by the operation of wider social relations/structures of power. Such an approach allows us to examine the internal and external power dynamics of policy networks, which may be particularly relevant where these networks are multiagency or interorganisational in nature. Unlike network analysis, which focuses on policy *formation*, moreover, Benson's approach may be particularly useful for understanding the operation of policy delivery or *implementation* networks and, indeed, for understanding the relationship between the two. This chapter sets out to apply the insights of both approaches to the child protection context. After describing the characteristics or 'architecture' of this complex policy area, the chapter will identify some of the key tensions that may be seen to characterise its operation.

The core policy community

At first sight the precise configuration of the child protection policy community appears elusive. The traditional focus of central government departments on functional areas (social services, education, health) rather than on specific groups of people (children and families, people with disabilities, older people) means that there is no single visible community with overall responsibility for ensuring the welfare of children and young people nor for producing the principles and standards for the development of relevant services. Policy responsibilities for children and young people are shared across a wide and diverse range of departments which, in varying combinations and on an intermittent and time-limited basis, may collaborate on specific policy issues that cut across their sectional domains. These departments may include those for Education and Employment (education, youth service, training), Social Security, the Environment (housing, local authorities), Defence (service family welfare), Culture, Media and Sport and that of the Lord Chancellor (family law). The Report of the National Commission of Inquiry into the Prevention of Child Abuse concluded that this was a problematic arrangement: "… the country has a set of co-operative arrangements between agencies whose main concerns range far more widely than the interest of children" (Mostyn, 1996, p 55). There was a need, it concluded, to bring a 'sharper focus' to the process of government by locating responsibility for children and young people 'firmly and publicly' in a single organisational form. While moves in this direction have been made in Wales by the appointment of a Children's Commissioner, no such development has yet taken place in England. On closer scrutiny, however, it is possible to identify a core organisational location for the development of child welfare and protection policy. More than any other single government department, the lead in developing a consistent approach to child protection and child welfare policy has been assumed (for England and, until its political devolution, Wales) by the Department of Health (DoH). Core policy responsibility for children's services lies with the Secretary of State for Health, although in practice this is discharged by a parliamentary Under-Secretary of State who is not a Cabinet minister. Within the DoH, child protection is located under one of two children's services branches of the Social Care Group (see Figure 2). Applying the Wilkes and Wright (1987) typology, child protection can be understood as a specific policy dimension of the 'children's services' sub-sector of the broader 'social care' policy sector, itself located under the overall policy area of 'health'.

Many commentators have argued that decision making in the DoH has traditionally been dominated by a closed and tight-knit 'iron triangle' of ministers, civil servants and representatives of the medical profession. Not only has an important role been played by external professional advisers, but also many of the department's civil servants themselves have traditionally had these professional backgrounds (Brown, 1975). As such, some contend, it may at times be more appropriate to view these groups as effectively 'internal' to the department (Richardson and Jordan, 1979). Ham (1999) suggests that the dominance of producer groups able to promote and defend their interests has meant that the DoH has engaged in strategies of appeasement and conflict resolution, with negotiation rather than consultation typically characterising the policy process. As a result, decision making has been incremental and conservative in nature, characterised by a largely negative approach to policy development: "... gatekeepers reduce the number of demands competing for the time and attention of policy-makers, and non-decision-making operates to rule some issues off the agenda" (Ham, 1999, p 127).

Some argue, however, that the political reforms of the NHS at the end of the 1980s effectively ended the 'producer capture' of the health policy process. In this view, the review of the service, encapsulated in *Working for patients* (DoH, 1989a), appeared to consolidate the power of the managers at the expense of the clinicians, moving doctors' organisations from the centre of health policy affairs to the 'pluralistic margins' (Salter, 1998, p 212). Rather than corporatist accommodation, Salter argues, by the end of the decade the initially amicable relationship between the four key power groups within the NHS – politicians, bureaucrats, managers and medics – had degenerated into "... a state of simmering tension" (p 21). Klein (1995), however, considers that the reforms did not radically shift the balance of power between these groups. While the autonomy of medics may have been eroded at a local level, nationally the ascendancy of the managers was constrained by the professional power of clinicians. What the reforms did do, however, was to prompt clinicians to take

Figure 2: Child protection framework

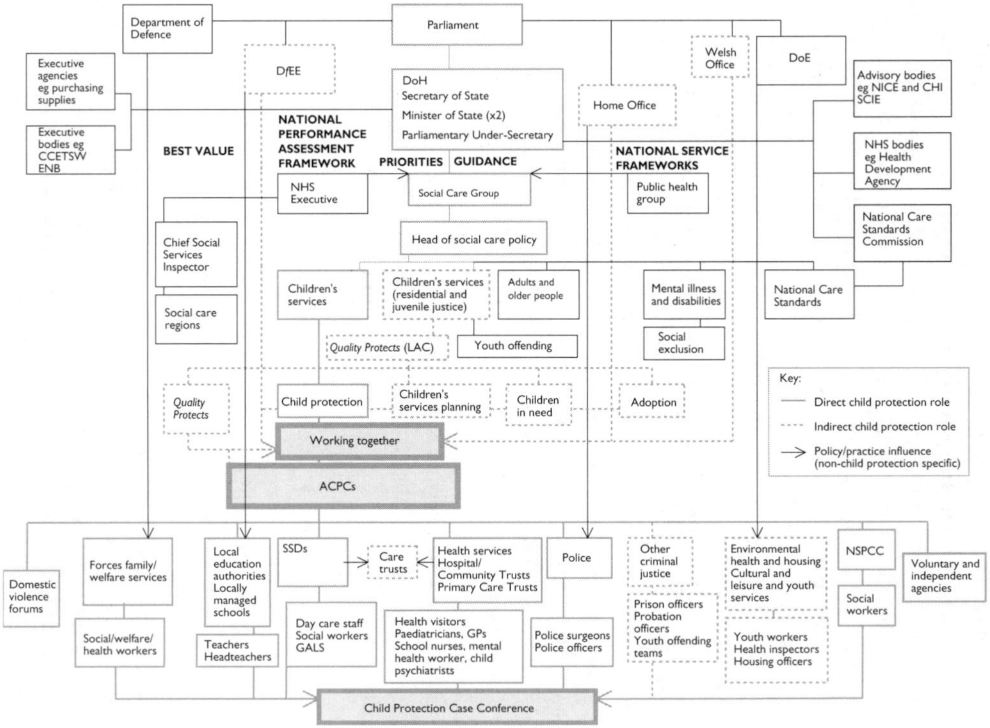

Notes:

CCETSW	Central Council for Education and Training in Social Work
CHI	Commission for Health Improvement
ENB	English National Board
GALS	Guardians ad Litem
LAC	Looked After Children
NICE	National Institute for Clinical Excellence
NSPCC	National Society for the Prevention of Cruelty to Children
SCIE	Social Care Institute for Excellence

Key:

— Direct child protection role

— Indirect child protection role

→ Policy/practice influence (non-child protection specific)

Parliament

Department of Defence

DfEE

DoH
Secretary of State
Minister of State (x2)
Parliamentary Under-Secretary

Home Office

Welsh Office

DoE

Advisory bodies eg NICE and CHI SCIE

NHS bodies eg Health Development Agency

National Care Standards Commission

National Care Standards

NATIONAL PERFORMANCE ASSESSMENT FRAMEWORK

BEST VALUE

PRIORITIES GUIDANCE

NATIONAL SERVICE FRAMEWORKS

Public health group

Mental illness and disabilities

Social exclusion

Adoption

NHS Executive

Social Care Group

Head of social care policy

Adults and older people

Youth offending

Children in need

Children's services

Children's services (residential and juvenile justice)

Children's services planning

Chief Social Services Inspector

Social care regions

Quality Protects (LAC)

Quality Protects

Child protection

Working together

ACPCs

Executive agencies eg purchasing supplies

Executive bodies eg CCETSW ENB

Police

Police surgeons Police officers

Other criminal justice

Prison officers
Probation officers
Youth offending teams

Environmental health and housing
Cultural and leisure and youth services

Youth workers
Health inspectors
Housing officers

Voluntary and independent agencies

NSPCC

Social workers

Health services
Hospital/ Community Trusts
Primary Care Trusts

Care trusts

Health visitors
Paediatricians, GPs
School nurses, mental health worker, child psychiatrists

Child Protection Case Conference

SSDs

Day care staff
Social workers
GALS

Local education authorities
Locally managed schools

Teachers
Headteachers

Forces family/ welfare services

Social/welfare/ health workers

Domestic violence forums

appropriate measures, by more active (self) performance monitoring, to pre-empt any further tightening of managerial control. Although as we write the implications of New Labour's reforms on the balance of power within the NHS have yet fully to play out, at least via the developments in primary care they appear to have restored the power of doctors relative to those of managers, albeit within a stronger regulatory framework imposed by central government: a situation of 'centrally controlled devolution' (Light, 1998; see Chapter Five for a more extended discussion of this issue).

The health policy sector, however, is not homogeneous; it comprises a number of different policy sub-sectors, characterised by a variety of policy-making communities and networks. In particular, these are likely to encompass the continuum of types described by Marsh and others, from the formal tight-knit consensual 'policy communities' at one end to the larger and looser 'issue networks' at the other (Marsh, 1998). Thus, for example, Haywood and Hunter's (1982) analysis of the NHS in the early 1980s contrasted the tight-knit 'iron triangles' seen to surround the older persons' policy community, with the looser 'issue networks' characteristic of policy development in areas such as health services organisation. The metaphor these authors used for the older person policy community of the early 1980s was that of a policy issue network with an iron triangle core, in which organisations in the 'outer circle' are essentially supportive of, and closely allied to, those in the inner circle. The cohesiveness of the core and outer networks was seen to derive from the need to compete for scarce resources with other more powerful sub-sector networks.

To an extent, Haywood and Hunter's model appears to be applicable to the child protection policy context. This similarly appears to be characterised by a small, hierarchical decision-making core operating within a more diverse, but fairly stable, wider issue network. The relationship between this inner core and the wider issue network, however, may be less close and consensual than that seen to characterise older persons' policy. Two interrelated tiers appear to be evident, but the uneven nature of their relationship may be such as to suggest that the child protection 'policy architecture' is characterised by a 'core-periphery' model. That is, a central policy community (with 'iron triangle' characteristics) closely linked to, but not embedded within, a more peripheral issue network. Although less consensual and more diverse than the core community, the involvement of the peripheral issue network is more stable than that of other interested or 'attentive parties' who may seek to influence the development of child protection policy.

The membership of the core policy community involves a restricted group of ministers, officials and representatives of professional/producer groups. In addition to officials from the DoH's Social Care Group, for example, the steering group for the 1999 *Working together* guidance involved representatives of key producer organisations – the Association of Directors of Social Services (ADSS), the Association of Chief Police Officers (ACPO) and the Local Government Association (LGA) – as well as one non-statutory agency, the National Society for the Prevention of Cruelty to Children (NSPCC). Other key interests, however, notably representatives of social or health professionals and, apart from the NSPCC, pressure groups for child or parental rights, are excluded from the core policy community. The relative political weakness of the British Association of Social Work (BASW) has meant that the core policy community has typically utilised individual academics, the ADSS and, to a lesser extent, the LGA, as a proxy for the social care professional perspective.

Frequently, although not routinely, the core community displays an intergovernmental dimension. Thus the *Working together* steering group also involved officials and ministers from the departments of Education and Employment and the Home Office as well as the National Assembly for Wales. Interdepartmental collaboration has characterised policy making in areas such as sex offenders, abuse of trust, vulnerable witnesses, as well as the development of good practice memoranda. Indeed, child protection policy may be unusual to the extent that it is a joint product of these different departments. Other areas of cross-sector policy initiatives are more typically developed by specific departments, working in conjunction with their colleagues elsewhere. Such was the 1998 Home Office-led Ministerial Group for the Family and the explicitly DoH-led *Quality Protects* framework developed in the same year.

In general this core policy community appears to operate on the basis of shared values and accepted legitimacy of outcome. The state or 'state actors' play a pivotal role and ensure that the community works closely to government (or Cabinet) requirements. The more limited involvement of social care professions compared with their medical counterparts lessens the need for the core community to engage in the strategies of appeasement and conflict resolution that characterise other aspects of NHS policy generation. The rift between the 'managers' and the 'mandarins' identified by Ham (1999), moreover, may be less apparent in the Social Care Group than in the other two business divisions of the department (NHS Executive and Public Health) given the lesser likelihood of service allegiance on the part of those with social care backgrounds. On the other hand, the potential for conflict remains, between the different producer groups involved, between these groups and the civil servants (and the politicians behind them) and between the representatives of local and central government. Although the power of local authorities has been constrained, they nevertheless remain an important layer between central policy and local practice. This role of 'intermediary' may represent a source of tension within the core policy community.

The intergovernmental dimension of the child protection community is task-specific and time-limited in nature, falling somewhere between the 'radical' and 'routinised' coordination described by Webb (1991). Whereas the latter is well established and taken for granted, the former implies change and disturbance: "... the crossing of boundaries between mutually exclusive, competitive or previously unrelated interests or domains" (Webb, 1991, p 231). Although underpinned by the inclusive approach of the 1989 Children Act, interdepartmental collaboration in child protection remains susceptible to potential conflicts of interest between participants with different policy agendas. Thus, for example, there may be tensions between the child welfare concerns of the DoH and the community safety/youth justice objectives of the Home Office or between the aim of enhancing social inclusion and the exclusive tendencies of the Department for Education and Employment's (DfEE's) educational marketplace.

There may also be potential for conflict between the child protection policy community, centred on the DoH, and other policy networks emerging in the late 1990s and early 2000s in the broad area of children's services, some of which may involve overlapping membership. In 2000, for example, a new Cabinet Committee on Children and Young People's Services was set up, chaired by the Chancellor of the Exchequer, with the Education Secretary as the vice-chair and involving the Ministers for Health, Defence and Culture. Working to this committee is a Children and Young Person's Unit, based at the DfEE, but chaired by a new Minister for Young People (Boateng), based at the Home Office and responsible for administering a new multi-million pound Children's Fund (see Chapter Six for further details). These initiatives were in addition to the existing Family Policy Committee, chaired by the Home Secretary, with a brief to develop policies to support families and underpin marriage. While the government has denied any conflict between these new committees and the role of the DoH, the new Minster for Young People has nevertheless made very clear his view of the need for a fresh approach to child welfare and protection issues (Rickford, 2000, p 21). At the very least, their existence may serve as a reminder of the importance of adhering closely to the government's policy agenda.

The peripheral issue network

In contrast to the close-knit nature of core policy communities, issue networks are defined (Marsh, 1998) as encompassing the full range of affected interests, with fluctuating membership and levels of contact. Although more heterogeneous than the core policy community, the child protection issue network nevertheless displays some predictability and continuity of membership. Longstanding players in this issue network include representatives of core professional groups (social workers, health professionals and teachers) and user groups/children's charities (Family Rights Group, Barnardo's, The Children's Society and so on) as well as those academic/policy researchers not utilised by the DoH as advisors or 'preferred providers'. Issue networks are, however, characterised by unequal degrees of involvement with, or access to, the core decision-making process on the part of their 'members'. Thus it is interesting to note, for example, that while the DoH undertook acknowledged collaboration with nursing and medical professional associations (Conference of Royal Medical Colleges, Standing Nursing and Midwifery Advisory Committee, BMA) in the production of the relevant addendum to *Working together*, no such formal role appears to have been played by representatives of social work or social care professionals.

The heterogeneous membership of an issue network moreover increases the possibility of disagreement and tension between its members. On many questions it is possible that a degree of consensus will emerge. The potential for conflict within a network of contrasting interests, however, is likely to be high. Unlike the core policy community, which is characterised by a rough balance of power, "… a positive-sum game" (Marsh, 1998, p 16), the operation of a typical issue network is characterised by the unequal power and resources of its members. Given this, the interests of some members are likely to be advanced at the expense of others (a 'zero-sum' game). The child protection network, for example, involves representatives of both service users and service providers and from organisations focusing on the rights of children as well as those promoting the rights of parents or families. The peripheral network also involves representatives of different professional groups, such as social workers and doctors, who may have very different strategic policy objectives.

The relationship between the core policy community and the wider issue network is essentially uneven. On the one hand, despite the different sectional interests by which it is constituted, the child protection policy area may be unusual in the extent of internal unanimity about the ultimate policy goals and, to a certain extent, about the means by which these goals are to be achieved. Few participants would disagree, for example, that protecting children from abuse or neglect requires more effective cooperation on the part of a wide range of agencies and professional groups at a local level. The high political sensitivity of the child protection issues also means that both core community and issue network tend to be united against the common threat of public/political opprobrium resulting from practice failure. Consultation between the policy core and the peripheral network moreover has been considerable. The development of the 1999 *Working together* guidance, for example, involved two separate rounds of consultation, drawing on "... the expertise of a wide range of experts" (DoH, 1999a).

On the other hand, the relationship between core and peripheral elements of the child protection policy framework is, potentially at least, also oppositional. Some of those in the wider issue network may feel resentment at being excluded from the heart of policy making and others may feel that their particular area of interest has been marginalised or ignored in the outcome of the policy process. Significant differences exist about, for example, the respective rights and responsibilities of children, their families and the state, the appropriate balance between prevention and protection and the acceptable degree of central prescription over the procedures surrounding child protection work. These all represent potential areas of tension within the wider issue network and between groups within the network and the core policy community. It is arguable, moreover, that some forms of consultation may serve more as a mechanism for legitimising decisions already taken by the core policy community than as a means of informing those decisions. Apart from some small changes, such as the time limit for child protection review conferences, for example, the difference between the first and final draft of the *Working together* document was noticeably slight. The second round of consultation indeed was something of a 'holding operation', designed to enable the associated consultation on the new Assessment Framework to catch up.

Local provider networks

A key link between policy development at the central level and its implementation at the local level is the Area Child Protection Committee

(ACPC). Established initially as Area Review Committees (ARCs) following the 1974 report into the death of Maria Colwell, and redesignated as ACPCs in 1988, the role of these bodies is to develop, monitor and review local systems for interagency cooperation in individual cases, including the production of local procedural handbooks or manuals. Although not involved in the management of individual cases, ACPCs are responsible for overseeing the 'Part 8' reviews undertaken in cases of child deaths, bringing together information from the management reviews undertaken in individual agencies. Despite their role in the coordination of interagency work, however, the ACPCs are not statutory bodies and have no executive role. As such they have no authority to compel constituent agencies to comply with the decisions they make. The representatives of the individual agencies that comprise the ACPCs are individually accountable to their respective organisations, which are held to be jointly accountable for the actions of the ACPCs.

Although the exact composition of the local ACPC is to be 'determined locally', the central policy community has provided fairly detailed recommendations about which agencies should be involved. Reflecting the gradual enlargement of the interagency base of child protection activity, as well as the fragmentation of health and social care services, the range of recommended member agencies has grown with each successive version of the official guidance. The initial recommendation for membership was for senior level representation from local and health authorities, police, probation and the NSPCC. By 1991 the list was much longer and more specific. In respect of the NHS, for example, explicit mention was made of the district health authorities (DHAs) and the then family health services authorities (FHSAs) as well as representation from nurses, hospital doctors, GPs (via the General Medical Committees) and psychiatric workers. Not all the agencies/professional groups listed in the guidance, however, have been equally involved in the work of the ACPCs. Research undertaken in the mid-1990s by Sanders et al (1997), for example, distinguished *full membership* of the committees, which they saw as only really exemplified by social services staff, from the *significant involvement* of the police and certain health professionals (for example, paediatricians) and the more *peripheral involvement* of others, such as education, probation and some health members (see Chapter Seven for a more extended discussion of the composition and role of the ACPCs).

The final tier of the child protection framework is that of individual casework by 'front-line' practitioners. In their day-to-day collaboration they make up the local *provider* or *delivery networks*. The multiagency and multidisciplinary nature of child protection work means that these networks involve a wide range of different professional groups. As with the ACPCs, however, not all groups may be equally involved. Hallett (1995) found evidence of a network operating on four interacting layers: social workers, police and paediatricians comprising the first 'core' layer; the second layer involving the more generic 'front-line' professions, such as health visitors, teachers and GPs, with day-to-day contact with children; followed by 'case-specific' professions such as lawyers, accident and emergency staff, psychologists and psychiatrists; and finally what Hallett and Birchall termed the more 'peripheral' professions with no formal responsibility for child or family care but who were occasionally used in advisory, consultative or pastoral roles, such as school nurses, education welfare officers and youth workers (Hallet, 1995, p 263). Again as with the ACPCs, successive versions of *Working together* have gradually extended the scope of the front-line network. The 1999 document encompasses all agencies working with children and young people, including the youth services, day care services, the youth justice service as well as adult services, such as mental health teams and substance misuse services, and calls on the full 'corporate capacity' of the local authority, including housing and leisure services (see Chapter Eleven for a more detailed discussion of the local provider networks).

Threats to collaboration

Marsh (1998) argues that the closer a network is towards the 'policy community' end of the spectrum, the greater its ability to ensure policy continuity and achieve desired policy change. The high political sensitivity of child protection has resulted in the perceived need for strong central scrutiny of policy development and implementation. The role of successive child abuse inquiries in shaping, not only the content of government policy, but the means or methods by which it is to be implemented, has been pivotal. Despite its apparent voluntarism, reflected in the lack of mandatory reporting, for example, the operation of the national child protection community has become increasingly *dirigiste*. The 'horizontal articulation' sought via (albeit time-limited) interdepartmental cooperation has been accompanied by a strong thrust towards tight vertical integration, or 'mandated cooperation' (Hallett, 1995) of the different layers of the child protection framework. Central to this cooperation, and to the close interrelationship of policy development and policy implementation, is the role of the central *Working together* guidance.

Child protection is a distinctive policy area in that the bulk of its procedures and practice derive not from primary legalisation, but from subsequent regulations, circulars of guidance and codes of good practice. In addition to the 10 volumes of accompanying guidance and regulation covering specific areas of the 1989 Children Act, a detailed operational framework for all central aspects of the interagency child protection process is provided by successive editions of the *Working together* guidance (DHSS and Welsh Office, 1988; Home Office et al, 1991; DoH et al, 1999). Subsequent addenda set out to clarify the roles of specific professional groups, such as nurses, health visitors and midwives (DoH and Standing Nursing and Midwifery Advisory Committee, 1997), doctors (DoH, 1996) and the health and education services more generally (DoH, 1995; WOC, 1995). Other circulars of guidance or memoranda of good practice have been produced to deal with particular issues such as disclosure of criminal backgrounds on those with access to children (Home Office, 1996), partnership working (DoH and SSI, 1995), guidelines for trainers and managers working with child sexual abuse (Doh and SSI, 1996) or video interviewing of child witnesses (Home Office and DoH, 1992).

The *Working together* guidance is officially defined as a statement of good practice which does not have the full force of statute, but "... should be complied with unless local circumstances indicate exceptional reasons which justify a variation" (DoH et al, 1999). As Sanders (1999) reports, however, the reality may be more complex: while non-compliance may leave an authority vulnerable to criticism or prosecution, at least one local authority has been challenged in the courts for attempting to comply with government guidance (not in this case the *Working together* guidance). Nevertheless, given the political sensitivity of the area and the limited public support given to the social work profession, considerable operational weight is attached to these circulars of guidance. The residual culture of voluntarism underpinning the English child protection system meant that the central policy community stopped short of itself developing specific practice protocols. Nevertheless, via the production of detailed proposals for activities such as assessment and case review and by the responsibility given to the ACPCs to develop common operational definitions and thresholds for intervention, it is arguable that the guidance has moved closer to mandating the *means* as well as the desired *ends* of multiagency child protection work. The result has been the accusation by some commentators that the child protection process has become overly 'proceduralised', leaving little room for professional discretion or innovation (for example, Parton, 1994).

Despite the increased degree of central prescription surrounding the work of local provider networks, threats to collaboration remain inherent within multiagency and interprofessional networks. As Benson has argued, agencies/professional groups function primarily to maintain and pursue their organisational self-interest (via defence of service paradigms, maintenance of scarce resources and establishment of legitimacy). Aspects of collaboration, or collaboration itself, may thus be resisted if seen to damage an organisation's 'market position'. A central concern of the *Working together* guidance is to encourage consensus on both *domain* (who does what) and *ideological* (how it is done) dimensions within local provider networks. Particularly within networks characterised by interprofessional collaboration, however, consensus around the appropriate means or methods of working may be difficult to achieve. As described in Chapter Three, the basis of professional power derives from the control over, and privileging of, certain types of knowledge. Resistance to sharing these with, or subordinating them to, those of professionals from different disciplinary areas remains a potential constraint on the achievement of effective interagency working. Domain and ideological consensus will also be affected by higher societal evaluation of certain types of knowledge (for example, medical rather than social). This will influence perceptions about the roles to be played by different network participants as well as affect judgements about appropriate methods of intervention.

Domain and ideological consensus within networks may also be hindered by different degrees of power and/or involvement on the part of its participants. The role played by a particular organisation within a multiagency network, for example, will be significantly affected by the nature of its links to wider structures of social, political or professional power. More powerful groups (such as medical professionals) may work to ensure that the terms of interorganisational exchange are such as to protect and enhance their dominance within the network. Relative power may also derive from the greater perceived centrality of some agencies (such as SSDs) to the operation of the network, as a result of their lead role in service delivery, for example, or the dominance of their service paradigms. In turn, domain inconsistencies may arise if not all those agencies participating perceive themselves equally central to the operation of the network. Less centrally involved agencies are likely to be less committed to the objectives of network activities and may remain more susceptible to the pull of alternative agendas.

Whatever the possibilities of encouraging ideological consensus on the part of network participants, it is difficult to legislate for the condition of *positive evaluation*. A range of factors can adversely affect the extent to which professional groups/agencies value each other's roles. These can be seen to operate at both interpersonal and interprofessional levels. At the interpersonal level, network relations can be affected by differences of race, sex, age and class. While difficult in themselves, these factors may become particularly problematic for interprofessional working when overlaid with differences in status and power. Thus, for example, the relative status and power of doctors vis-à-vis nurses has been interwoven with the 'gendered' nature of the professional groups involved (Kendrick, 1995). Interprofessional stereotyping may also negatively affect relationships within an interagency network, with such stereotyping being more likely to occur when particular groups of professionals come together only infrequently (Blyth and Milner, 1990). Such difficulties may be particularly relevant to the operation of child protection networks, given the sheer range and diversity of the professional groups and agencies involved.

In addition to tensions arising from lack of domain/ideological consensus and limited positive evaluation, the operation of child protection provider networks may also be affected by problems of *work coordination*. The existence of different patterns of work organisation within the many agencies/groups involved may make it logistically difficult for them to collaborate at either strategic or operational levels. Particular areas of tension may derive from variations in work and caseload management. Thus it may be difficult for professional groups to collaborate effectively when some (such as general practitioners/teachers) have to work around fixed contact hours (surgery/classroom/clinic) and others, such as social workers, appear to have more flexible working arrangements. Professional groups and agencies also differ importantly in respect of the forms of governance and accountability to which they are subject. Tensions may arise, for example, between agencies (such as social services departments [SSDs] which are primarily accountable to their local electorates, those (such as health authorities) which are ultimately accountable to central government, and others (such as medics) who may see themselves as primarily accountable to their professional associations. Yet other difficulties may arise as a result of the different extent to which member agencies have decentralised their decision-making structures. Some front-line staff (such as GPs) may be in a position to make decisions on issues that others (such as teachers) would have to refer up to line managers.

Finally, equilibrium within child protection delivery networks may be particularly susceptible to the impact of external organisational change, again due to the sheer range of agencies involved. The radical restructuring of the public sector, for example, that occurred during the 1980s and 1990s affected not just the structures of service provision, but also the ideology or ethos by which they were underpinned. For local child protection networks, the development of internal markets within health and social care and the process of local government reorganisation may have been particularly problematic, disturbing established contacts and systems. The impact of these changes, moreover, is likely to have been worsened by the variable and uneven way in which they affected different agency and professional participants. Arguably, one reason for the extremely detailed practice framework characterising child protection has been the recognition that the process of external change introduces new uncertainties into interagency collaboration.

Conclusion

This chapter has attempted to set out the key characteristics of the child protection policy framework. Using the models of network theory, it has argued that this framework involves a combination of different network types and layers. At the national level, policy development is characterised by the routine collaboration of a small tight-knit and fairly exclusive policy community, comprising ministers, officials and selected professional and academic advisors. Periodically, this small community expands into a wider intergovernmental network in order to agree specific policy and practice guidelines. While the operation of the core community appears predominantly consensual, not least given the limited power of the provider interests involved, threats to cohesion are introduced by the engagement of other central government departments or networks with different, and possibly conflicting, policy objectives.

The politically sensitive nature of child protection requires that the core policy community operates effectively within a wider issue network encompassing the full range of affected groups, particularly those whose interests can be seen to be excluded from that core community. Although less cohesive and consensual than the core community, this network is more stable and predictable than any ad hoc collection of 'interested parties', with longstanding involvement by key service user and professional interest groups. However, the relationship between the core community and the peripheral issue network is uneven. Although sharing a broad consensus about the overall aims of child protection policy, potential or actual areas of conflict may arise around the means of achieving these aims and the assumptions by which they are underpinned. Interaction with the core policy community, moreover, is intermittent and may more typically be focused on the details rather than the broad brush of policy.

At the front-line level, the implementation of central policy objectives is undertaken by a series of local provider or delivery networks, working within the detailed framework for 'mandated coordination' established by the central policy community. The implementation of central directives, however, is never a simple matter; the gap between policy ambitions and their attainment at local levels has long been identified as a key policy problem (Barrett and Fudge, 1981; Ham and Hill, 1984). Potential barriers to effective collaboration within local provider networks are posed by a range of internal and external factors threatening ideological/domain consensus, work cooperation and/or mutual positive evaluation on the part of its participants. Two factors centrally influencing the internal dynamics of child protection provider networks are the different forms of accountability surrounding their organisational participants and the different disciplinary skills or 'knowledge domains' underpinning the work of their constituent professional groups. The following two chapters consider these aspects in greater depth.

THREE

Knowledge and networks

Introduction

This chapter and the next seek to understand why securing compliance with the 'cooperation mandate' in child protection may continue to be problematic. One of the major problems identified in successive child abuse inquiry reports (DHSS, 1982; DoH, 1991) was the failure of professionals to share vital knowledge and skills. A new approach to practice emerged as a result, based on the twin assumptions that knowledge in child protection could be standardised into written procedures and that children would be protected as long as professionals based their decisions on these knowledge 'stratagems'. This approach, however, posits a simplistic relationship between knowledge and its application. Drawing on theories of knowledge management, this chapter argues that the relationship between knowledge acquisition and human behaviour is complex. As such, it questions whether the introduction of knowledge stratagems such as practice protocols is sufficient to ensure effective interprofessional collaboration.

The chapter begins by considering the general tension between professional 'ways of knowing' and the attempt to codify this knowledge into detailed procedures that seek to influence, even control, professional action. It then examines the difficulties within interagency and interprofessional networks that may arise from the different, and at times competing, knowledge 'domains' of the various participants. The constraints over knowledge sharing are explored and the chapter considers the ways in which the propensity to share can be disturbed by external factors such as organisational change and wider 'knowledge shifts'. A central concern is to illuminate the main factors that may serve to undermine the efficacy of knowledge stratagems as a means of controlling professional practice and ensuring network equilibrium.

Professional learning and social control

In the current political climate surrounding the public sector, demands for better evaluation of services, particularly of their 'value for money', have grown. These have been augmented by the desire for greater certainty, seeking solutions to variation in professional performance and service outcome. The next chapter highlights the ways in which the introduction of new public management (NPM) approaches to health and social care services attempted to 'open up' areas of professional practice to managerial scrutiny and control. These developments also sought to encourage the 'scientification' of professional practice by privileging the role of empirical 'evidence' over professional experience or intuition. Increasingly over the last years of the 1990s, there was an attempt to introduce into social care the 'evidence-based' practice seen to characterise the health care professions (Currey et al, 1993; Barnett, 1994). For many of its proponents, moreover, understanding 'what works' in social care practice is seen to require the experimental designs of natural scientific inquiry (Macdonald and Roberts, 1995; Sheldon, 1998).

These developments have two important, interrelated implications for professional practice. One is the assumption that professional knowledge can be codified into sets of rules and relationships that can be generalised across different situations and into other fields of work. The second is that the promotion of rule-based behaviour rests heavily on the presumption of technical rationality – that having received the relevant knowledge, the user will make rational choices between alternative courses of action, based on the anticipated consequences. There are, however, a number of potential weaknesses in both these assumptions that may be of particular relevance to our understanding of the role of professional knowledge in child protection networks.

The first is that, even when professionals are aware of the existence of written procedures, they may not always be willing or able to follow them. Suchman (1987), for example, has argued that individual actions are taken in the context of particular, concrete circumstances. Without knowing these circumstances, it is impossible to predict the outcome of these 'situated actions'. A statement of intent can thus say very little about the action that follows: "... the relationship of the intent to accomplish some goal to the actual course of situated action is enormously contingent" (1987, p 38). Typically we can only know what will happen once we are engaged in the action itself: "... it is frequently only acting in a present situation that makes its possibilities clear, and we often do not know ahead of time, or at least with any specificity what future states we desire to bring about" (p 38). Understanding the relationship between knowledge and action requires insight into the ways in which people's motivations, abilities and experience influence how they interpret events and so create the meaning that triggers action (Collins, 1990; Lave and Wenger, 1991).

Psychological approaches emphasise the extent to which absorbing, valuing, retaining and sharing knowledge are learned behaviours. Whether in a work context, or in personal relationships, people bring with them habitual responses based on their personal experiences that can either lead to more openness and honesty or to defensiveness and dishonesty (Fletcher and Fitness, 1996). As Schutz and Luckmann (1973) argue, the role of intuition and experience is important to the way people interpret events: "Meaning is the result of my explanation of past lived experience which is grasped reflectively from an actual now and from an actually valid reference schema" (1973, p 16). Organisational and occupational cultures and, on a broader level, the norms and values of the society in which people live, critically bear on the process of meaning creation.

Arguably, the relativistic, and to some extent idiosyncratic, processes of sense making and action taking limit the impact of standardised prescriptions imposed from 'outside'. This may be particularly the case in the specific context of child protection services. In many ways, the rule-based behaviour promoted by the 'what works' model appears to resonate with the dominant approach to child protection practice. As Howe (1992) argues, the "... translation of the problem of child abuse into an arrangement of monitoring and surveillance procedures", has privileged the view that services can be improved (and professionals can be protected) so long as practitioners are prepared to 'go by the book' (pp 505-7). The simultaneous call for professional assessment of abuse to be based on 'hard' forensic evidence has also added to the attraction of the evidence-based approach. Attention is called to cases where clear evidence exists, at the expense of cases where abuse may be probable, but impossible to prove.

On the other hand, many have argued (Parton et al, 1997; Buckley, 1999; Sarangi, 1998) that enduring social problems like child abuse are not always presented in ways that are easily definable or measurable. The often imprecise or contested nature of the knowledge about child protection, exemplified by the controversy over anal dilation theory (Blumenthal, 1994), compounds the difficulty of applying 'text-book' presentations (Sarangi, 1998, p 241). In these circumstances, it is argued, professionals think 'in action' (Schon, 1983), relying on the skills of reflective, intuitive and experience-based practice rather than on standardised solutions imposed from outside. Buckley's (1999) study of social work decision making in child protection highlights the centrality of personal beliefs and values in making sense of the available information. Buckley also found that this 'sense making' was often based on very pragmatic concerns such as keeping workloads manageable. Given this, Richey and Roffman (1999) have argued that the implementation of externally imposed guidelines in the field will always involve some degree of 'tinkering' by practitioners who strive to accommodate the standard prescriptions with the unique factors surrounding a particular case.

Arguably, there are two other important areas of weakness with approaches that seek to codify professional knowledge and promote rule-based behaviour. One is the assumption that people are highly motivated to accept what others suggest 'works'. Another is that presenting evidence as objective, value-free 'truth' serves to camouflage the intellectual 'power relations' that underpin knowledge acquisition and sharing in inter-professional, multidisciplinary contexts. Accepting that something 'works' may centrally depend on the social status of those promoting or undertaking the action involved. In the next section we look at how the evaluation of various types of knowledge, and decisions about whether to make this knowledge available to others, is bound up with issues of professional power and organisational culture.

Professional knowledge domains and boundaries

A number of commentators have argued that the individual agency level of decision making cannot be disentangled from conceptual frameworks reflecting organisational priorities and the broader structures of social and political power (Fairclough, 1989; Giddens, 1991; Smith, 1993). A professional trained within a specific discipline will draw on on a distinctive knowledge base (Ouchi, 1980; Bernstein, 1990; Klein, 1996). When practitioners from different disciplines are brought together to address a particular social problem, there is likely to be divergence on a number of different dimensions. For example, we can expect that a particular professional group will apply a certain frame of reference, will highlight particular types of information as evidence of abuse and will categorise this information according to their distinctive professional (explicit and implicit) encoding system. Professionals in other fields are likely to utilise different reference points, creating the potential for misunderstanding or disagreement. As Whittington (1983) notes, there is a tendency for occupational groups: "... to develop a language which is meaningful to the group but [which is] jargon or impressive mystery to outsiders" (1983, p 268).

Competition between different knowledge domains is possible when there are different ideological, cultural or professional-specific approaches to the problem. It is also possible to the extent that professional power (and thus wealth creation) is based on claims to the unique possession of knowledge (Fairclough, 1989; van Dijk, 1997). Writing about the professional dominance of clinicians in the health service, for example, Friedson (1970) suggests that 'occupation closure' (denying access to other groups) is the central strategy to maintain professional boundaries and power. In order to safeguard professional power, status and identity certain forms of knowledge may not be made available to other professional groups. Claims to expert knowledge also depend on their acceptance by society at large. Securing and maintaining professional power requires public approval for appropriately certificated individuals to use their 'art and craft' in the solution of complex problems. In professions like medicine, application of this art and craft requires being able to convince the public of its altruistic nature. It also requires an ability to present the essentially subjective use of professional judgement as a form of objectivity. As Alvesson (1993, p 1000) argues, the 'myths of technocracy' serve to maintain the powerful mystique surrounding dominant professions like medicine. Interestingly, of course, despite their claim to objective science, medical professionals are among those most likely to resist the attempts to codify professional knowledge involved in the 'evidence-based' approach. Centrally prescribed, 'top-down' knowledge stratagems that seek to promote rule-based behaviour may be perceived by many professionals as a form of bureaucratisation and an unjustifiable constraint on professional autonomy (this argument is explored more fully in the next chapter).

The way in which knowledge is acquired and shared is also shaped by the culture of the organisation within which professionals work. Bair (1997) describes three types of organisational cultures which display different approaches to knowledge sharing:

- The *balkanised* organisations, with multiple 'warlords' competing against each other in an atmosphere of mutual suspicion and information hoarding. The potential for knowledge sharing is low here.
- The *monarchies*, characterised by authoritarian rule, where knowledge

tends to be passed 'top-down'. The potential for knowledge sharing is better here than in the 'balkans' but is still low.
• The *federations*, with local autonomy, a global framework and a civil form of dispute resolution. Cooperation is based on enlightened self-interest and the potential for sharing knowledge is high.

When knowledge sharing is not built into organisational processes, Bair concludes, when it is not seen as a normal and expected part of daily working life, it is unlikely to occur.

It could be argued that decision making in the NHS most closely resembles the 'monarchy' model, with doctors and health managers sitting at the top and nursing and health care workers at the lower levels. The literature on inter- and intra-professional relationships in health (Strauss et al, 1963; Friedson, 1970; Mackay and Webb, 1993; Kendrick, 1995) highlights the gendered and hierarchical social relationships that underlie the division of knowledge in medicine. This division is accentuated by subject and disciplinary specialisms and by the struggle of more 'marginal' professions such as nursing to gain professional status (Chan and Rudman, 1998). Klein describes how the divisive nature of professional boundaries reinforces the hierarchical ordering of (and reward for) different knowledge claims:

> The rhetoric of boundaries is signified by spatial metaphors of turf, territory and domain. Metaphors of place call attention to the ways categories and classifications stake out differences. Boundary work is the composite set of claims, activities and institutional structures that define and protect knowledge practices. As legitimacy and authority are attached to this knowledge, reputational systems are created and knowledge becomes hierarchically stratified. (Klein, 1996, p 1)

Clearly, the existence of professional boundaries can inhibit knowledge sharing. Change to these boundaries, however, in so far as it encourages defensiveness, may also be destructive to collaborative working. Boundaries, of course, also exist in a spatial sense in that professionals may not have much contact with professionals in other workplaces. The need for face-to-face contact in fostering interprofessional working has been highlighted in a number of studies (Davenport and Prusack, 1998; Wensley, 1998), with Davenport and Prusack revealing that professionals exchange knowledge in direct proportion to the level of personal contact.

Tensions around professional knowledge domains and boundaries may be especially acute in the child protection context. Where there is little agreement about the nature of the phenomenon, consensus around that nature of the 'evidence' may be particularly difficult to achieve. Thus Sarangi (1998) finds that doctors working with a medical model of child abuse tend to disclose only what they see as 'hard' evidence (for example, physical signs or symptoms), while social work professionals undertaking comprehensive assessments are more inclined to assess risk on the basis of circumstantial evidence. In this way the status of the evidence can affect how and whether it is communicated: "The issue of what information is reportable to whom and by whom thus becomes entangled with the very status of such information (whether it is evidential or circumstantial)" (Sarangi, 1998, p 251). Power relations between professionals can thus have an influential role in the establishment of what is and what is not a 'fact' (Atkinson, 1995), with the credibility of particular information being linked to the status of its source. As Sarangi puts it: "... who makes a claim is as important as the claim itself" (1998, p 245).

Dominant professional groups like doctors, moreover, can play an important gatekeeping role in terms of selecting or endorsing information for particular purposes (Goffman, 1974). This can work to disregard or 'silence' information that may be seen as a potential threat, particularly if the informant is perceived to be of an inferior status. Thus, for example, the Jasmine Beckford inquiry found that the (in retrospect crucial) views of the female health visitor were ignored in favour of those expressed by the male doctors involved (London Borough of Brent, 1985). Sheppard (1995) found that GPs tend to be reluctant to initiate contact with more subordinate members of the health care team or with social services staff, perceiving that this is not their responsibility. Their expectation was that, as the head of health care teams, they should be kept informed by other team professionals (see Chapter Eight for further discussion of the role of the general practitioner in child protection).

The external environment

The ability to acquire and share knowledge is likely to be particularly poor in situations of organisational change, especially when professionals do not feel in control. Change strategies risk running into the problem of professional defensiveness or inertia as well as triggering more immediate human reactions of anxiety and insecurity. The mechanisms of public sector management and regulation challenge the notion that professionals are the experts who know what is best for the client. Such a context, it has been argued, diminishes the degree of control exercised by individual professionals (Gabe et al, 1994; Dominelli, 1996). As the next chapter indicates, some professional groups, like doctors, have been more successful than others in resisting bureaucratic or managerial forms of control. Generally it is clear that the boundaries of professional autonomy have been eroded by pressure for greater responsiveness to the consumer within the health and social care marketplace. Greater exposure to public scrutiny, however, can also result in professional protectionism. Thus, for example, there is evidence that increased public debate about the role of medical evidence in child protection has caused doctors to exercise greater caution in their clinical assessment due to concerns about possible recrimination (Hoyte, 1996).

In addition to the encroachment on professional decision making, the uncertainty often caused by organisational restructuring can impact on the capacity to learn and share new knowledge. There is some evidence that the preoccupation with survival in the face of job insecurity, rising workloads and the bureaucratisation of jobs like social work and education, impacts at the cognitive level by leaving practitioners too stressed or 'burnt-out' to apply their knowledge or absorb new information. Powell (1999), for example, highlights how the difficult financial context surrounding local authority SSDs may cause social workers to compromise agency procedures or professional values, in order to respond to the increasingly crisis-driven nature of their work. Morrison (1997) likewise argues that organisational restructuring, coupled with the often circumstantial nature of child protection concerns and the emotional nature of the work, can create an anxious working environment for practitioners. In this context, coping strategies can lead to the distortion of knowledge through feelings of defensiveness, resistance to sharing information and an unwillingness to reflect adequately on practice: "Emotional defensiveness ... deepens into cognitive distortion whereby the painful reality is warded off via denial of dissonant information and attitudes, offering a temporary but false sense of security" (Morrison, 1997, p 197).

Another layer of the 'anxious environment' for many professionals in the health and social care setting is the competitive culture of public sector markets. Many studies have highlighted the way that a competitive environment can foster knowledge hoarding in order to gain market advantage (Reich, 1991; Ives, et al, 1998; Aldridge, 1999). A competitive market culture may also militate against collaboration, especially if this is between agencies that are in effect rivals for the scarce resources of money and authority (Benson, 1975). More widely, it is likely that changing social attitudes will also have a significant bearing on professional knowledge domains. Thus, evolving public views about what constitutes child abuse and what should be done about it have been an important factor in challenging the knowledge base of particular professions and in changing the balance of disciplinary power between different professional groups.

Parton's (1985) charting of the politics of child abuse in the UK reveals how medicine, rather than social science, was critical in establishing the foundation of a generalisable knowledge. The medical profession played a vital role in identifying the physical signs of abuse through new scientific methods, such as x-ray technology, and in defining child abuse as a socio-medical condition, or 'syndrome', resulting from the psychopathology of individual parents. Parton also reveals how the impetus given to the role of medicine in child abuse was heightened by professional self-interest in the elevation of particular specialisms. Paediatric radiology, for example, occupied a relatively marginal status in medicine until the discovery of unexplained skeletal injuries through advances in x-ray technology offered an opportunity for the specialty to form coalitions with other more prestigious disciplines. Paediatrics had also been sliding to the margins of the medical profession before the discovery of the 'battered baby' syndrome provided a means of re-establishing its status: "The discovery of the battered baby could be seen to reinforce paediatrics in a crucial life-saving area of work which might help it to attract resources and re-establish its previous status" (Parton, 1985, p 58).

The growth of the paediatricians' interest in child abuse supports the argument of Gusfield (1989) that the claim for territory by a professional group rests on its ability to secure 'ownership' of a particular phenomenon: "To 'own' a social problem is to possess the authority to name that condition a 'problem' and to suggest what might be done about it" (Gusfield, 1989, p 433). The focus on the signs of physical abuse which could be empirically observed strengthened the expertise of the doctor as central to its diagnosis and treatment (Kempe and Kempe, 1978). The high status that medics such as paediatricians were to assume within the interprofessional multidisciplinary network was thus based on their 'knowledgeability'. This had an important impact on their relationships with practitioners from professional groups perceived to have less knowledge (and therefore status). The medicalisation of child abuse also drew attention away from alternative conceptualisations that linked it to poverty or the failure of political institutions. This limited the possibilities for other professional groups, such as welfare and community workers, to take a more active role in child protection.

During the late 1980s, the politicisation of child abuse, prompted by a number of high-profile cases, shifted concern from the prevention and treatment of child abuse to the identification and investigation of its occurrence. This development was reflected in a change of vocabulary within policy discourse from *child abuse* to *child protection*. It also had the effect of promoting 'investigative' rather than therapeutic practice and reconfigured the balance of power between different professional groups. As Parton explains:

> If in the past, child abuse has been seen as essentially a medico-social problem, where the expertise of the doctor has been seen as focal, increasingly it has been seen as a socio-legal problem, where legal expertise takes pre-eminence. (1991, p 18)

This new approach has not, however, been accompanied by any shift from the dominant assumption that child abuse results from individual failing (in parents/guardians) to acceptance of the role of social structural issues. Rather, it has been experienced more as a move from dealing with 'sickness' to dealing with 'villains and victims' (Gusfield, 1989, p 437).

Growing questions about the professional judgement of paediatricians also enabled the shift towards a more investigative/legalistic approach to child protection work. The Cleveland controversy and the foundation of PAIN (Parents Against Injustice) in the mid-1980s demonstrated a greater preparedness on the part of the public to question the validity of paediatric diagnoses, as well as those of other medical experts such as psychiatrists. In recent years, there has been further movement in the debate about child protection. Criticism from children and family pressure groups about the investigative, or adversarial, nature of child protection interventions, combined with the publication of two influential reports (*Child protection: Messages from research*, DoH, 1995a; *Childhood matters*, Mostyn, 1996), which argued for child abuse to be understood in the context of children's wider welfare needs. The resultant shift in service provision from child protection to family support and children in need – the 'lighter touch' – was reflected in the government's new *Framework for the assessment of children in need and their families* (DoH et al, 2000).

In this way, the developments in child protection reveal how the knowledge domains or 'territories' that professions seek to establish are relationships within interprofessional and multidisciplinary networks. When certain social issues appear to advance professional esteem, engagement with them may be sought after; conversely, when they bring the risk of professional or public opprobrium, involvement may be avoided. Arguably, in the politically sensitive context in which child protection cases are increasingly framed, coupled with the greater uncertainty surrounding their knowledge base, many in the medical profession (as well as other professional groups) may be increasingly disinclined to accord high priority to involvement in child protection work. General practitioners, for example, have often been accused by other professional groups of abrogating their child protection responsibilities (Hallett, 1995; Lupton et al, 1999b) and may not be alone in a perceived 'disowning' of child protection work. Thus Lupton et al's (1999b) study of local child protection networks revealed that paediatricians considered that orthopaedic surgeons, who have an important role in identifying skeletal injuries, were eschewing their responsibilities:

> "The orthopaedic surgeons don't want to know, so they don't deal with it as they don't like it." (named doctor, hospital paediatric ward, case study site, Lupton et al, 1999b, p 68)

Conclusion

The development of common practice guidelines or performance protocols is underpinned by the assumption that what professionals should know and what they should do can be captured in textual form and acquired through a formal learning process. The issues discussed presented in this chapter, however, suggest that the transition from 'knowing' to 'doing' is a complex and unpredictable process, affected by a range of factors at the individual, group and social level. The chapter also indicates that professional practice is characterised by other forms of knowledge and ways of learning that are not easily captured in knowledge stratagems and which can often place limits on the scope for interprofessional, multidisciplinary working. The attempt to mandate cooperation between professional groups via the development of practice protocols may thus underestimate the complex disciplinary dynamics embedded in interprofessional child protection work.

The achievement of consensus on 'domain' (who does what) and 'ideology' (how it is done) has been identified as central to the equilibrium, and therefore the effectiveness, of interorganisational networks. The foregoing discussion, however, indicates that the self-referent and context-sensitive nature of professional knowledge may make it difficult, and in some contexts impossible, to achieve consensus on these dimensions. 'Top-down' prescriptions for common practice may be particularly ineffective in so far as they assume the transfer of shared meanings across organisational and professional boundaries. As this chapter highlights, threats to network equilibrium are presented by such actions as 'knowledge hoarding', professional defensiveness and/or disciplinary 'turf wars'. Domain and ideological consensus can also fragment as a result of external factors. Thus, the changing discourse of child protection has influenced the balance of power between different professional groups within the local provider networks. In particular, the 'legalisation' and proceduralisation of child protection work has diminished the role of certain professional groups such as GPs and paediatricians, relative to that of social workers, lawyers and the police. The more recent policy shift towards family support and a 'lighter touch' does not appear significantly to have altered this situation.

The limits on directing collaboration from 'above' may also be exacerbated by tensions between different professional groups arising from their varying social and professional power. Thus, we have argued that the ability to define the nature of a social problem and to identify 'what works' in its treatment, is related to the social standing of the professional groups involved. Also centrally affecting the process of knowledge sharing and acquisition within networks are different organisational cultures and administrative structures (forms of governance, regulation and accountability) surrounding the practice of different professional groups (and the agencies within which they work). There may be particular problems, for example, with knowledge transfer in 'monarchies' or 'balkanised' organisations. The procedures of new public management (NPM), moreover, which have sought to increase the transparency of professional practice and its susceptibility to external regulation and control, have not affected all professional groups equally. Professional network participants differ crucially in terms of the extent to which they are susceptible to the state's regulatory capacity and the extent to which managerialist forms of accountability are balanced against, or resisted by, the perceived requirements of professional or democratic forms of accountability. The next chapter examines the issue of accountability in more depth and considers the extent to which differences between professionals and agencies in this respect have served to undermine the equilibrium of the child protection provider networks.

FOUR

Accountability, agencies and professions

Introduction

In the preceding chapters we have favoured Benson's 'interorganisational' approach as potentially the most helpful in explaining relationships within child protection networks (1975, 1983). We argue that his insistence that these relationships, theorised in four interrelated dimensions (*domain consensus*, *ideological consensus*, *positive evaluation* and *work coordination*), are not context-free but are rooted in 'sub-structural' influences, fits well with empirical evidence concerning provider networks in child protection. Benson's theory, however, is relatively silent on the role of the state in orchestrating policy implementation or in defining the parameters of acceptable practice surrounding interorganisational cooperation. In the case of child protection provider networks, the state's 'presence' relates most obviously to the dimension of work coordination (via regulatory and performance frameworks) although this is also mediated by the attributes of the three other dimensions. Benson's particular contribution, the identification of sub-structural factors (*external power/interests* and/or the *motivations of 'parent' organisations*) as determinants of the superstructural level, is germane to this chapter's focus on accountability. We suggest that the differing ability of provider agencies and professionals to resist the state's regulatory capacity (in both democratic and managerial forms) is important in understanding their engagement in child protection processes and that this can be explained with reference to substructural elements.

Network theory as proposed by Rhodes and Marsh (1992; Marsh, 1998) is of limited help since it focuses on 'meso' or 'apex' level relationships. The participation of professional groups in the core policy community assumes their members' support for the decisions they make. This arrangement, however, is insufficient to explain the failures or success of policy implementation, as regulation by explicit rules and guidelines also shapes policy at the level of practice. However, these mechanisms cannot be taken for granted. They are both fallible and at times contradictory, as agencies and professionals have different interests and obligations. In the case of professionals these obligations may variously be to the employer (for example, a trust), agency (NHS or local authority), profession or society. As there are clear differences in the susceptibility of different professions to the regulatory state, it is important to explore the complexities of accountability, its functionality to the modern state and the reasons why different accountability frameworks operate for different professional groups.

This chapter will explore the concept of accountability in its different modes and their operationalisation within the welfare state. In the local implementation of child protection policies, professional accountability to peers and to clients is traditionally seen to be important in determining standards of performance. However, professional accountability is not the only regulatory means sanctioned by society. Forms of democratic and managerial accountability are also of relevance as the state attempts to realise policies through increasingly complex and fragmented systems of governance. These different forms of accountability should be seen as overlapping rather than discrete, although not always convergent or mutually supportive. For example, an open system of managerial accountability should reinforce democratic accountability, but accountability to the client may be contradicted by accountability to the organisation.

The relative significance of the different forms of accountability in the regulation of the welfare state is not constant, but is context dependent. History, professional power and wider political and social events are all influential. In discussing the different forms of accountability, therefore, the chapter will explore why some professional groups in some contexts have been more successful than others in maintaining the primacy of peer accountability at the expense of bureaucratic forms of accountability. The significance of professional self-regulation will be considered in relation to the ability of medicine, nursing and social work to resist external regulatory regimes, thereby arguably undermining the possibility of more robust mechanisms of accountability. Similarly, in describing the histories of democratic and managerial (bureaucratic) modes of accountability, the chapter will identify the political rationale behind them. First the concept of accountability is explored.

The nature of accountability

Accountability is integral to social and political relationships. Without it, institutions would cease to function and the contract between state and citizen, on which civilised society is based, would fracture. The concept is simple enough: accountability is to be required to give an account for one's actions and to be held to account for those actions by others (Stewart, 1992; Day and Klein, 1997). It implies a delegation of power by those in authority to those sanctioned to carry out the duty. Accountability within markets is enforced in the first instance by contracts and then reinforced by law. Political accountability is more oblique. Governments are authorised to exercise power on behalf of the people and are held to account through the electoral system. However, ensuring accountability for the execution of government policies – in theory the blueprint broadly mandated by the electorate – is a more complex affair and one which, some argue, has become more problematic as a result of the 'differentiated polity' (Stewart, 1992; Weir and Hall, 1994) of the modern democratic state (see Chapter One).

The principles underpinning political accountability that Mill (1993) described in the 19th century – transparency, indivisibility and the power to hold to account[1] – were transferred to the extended state. They formed part of a moral agenda on which civil administration was to be based and which was ultimately embedded in parliamentary accountability. The growth of the state's welfare responsibilities, including those given to local authorities, was matched by more complex administrative arrangements. In the UK the development of the welfare state combined both bureaucratic and professional forms of power (Newman and Clarke, 1994). These derived from over-optimistic Fabian assumptions about the contribution that professional expertise could make to the solution of society's problems and the need for its rational coordination on a large scale. A specific form of organisational coordination emerged within the welfare state: the 'bureau-professional regime'. Newman and Clarke (1994) note that professionalism and bureaucracy are distinctive modes of power which are legitimated differently (by expertise and neutrality respectively), involve alternative modes of accountability and construct different relationships with those who receive welfare state services (clients, patients, customers, service users and so on). Critically, for an understanding of the differences in accountability and regulation experienced by the various professionals involved in child protection work, they also involve differences in the balance of power between professional and bureaucratic regimes in specific contexts. We begin with an exploration of professional accountability since the ability to assert its pre-eminence as a regulatory mechanism helps a profession to resist other forms of accountability.

Professional accountability

Operating a regime of professional accountability (being judged by one's peers) is a central pillar in the construction or maintenance of an autonomous profession. This is justified by the claim that professional practice was a sufficiently esoteric synthesis of knowledge and skills to be beyond the capacity of the layperson to assess (Etzioni, 1969). Professional accountability and autonomous decision making on behalf of the client, rather than the state, are regarded as key tenets of professional practice. Consequently, regulation by way of professional codes and a system of professional accountability has been a goal of those occupations aspiring to professional status.

This was achieved by the medical profession in the last century, and the last 30 years have seen the drive for professionalisation by both nursing and social work (Parry and Parry, 1979; Salvage, 1988). There has not, however, been universal support for this ambition in either occupation. Some dissenting voices have regarded professionalisation as an elitist strategy invoking class and racial discrimination (Cross, 1987, cited by Salvage, 1988) and creating barriers between carer and recipient. Others have seen it as using mystifying therapeutic approaches to enhance the controlling functions (of social work) (Jones, 1983, cited in Hugman, 1991). Unlike nursing, social work has long been divided over the need for a central council to regulate the conduct of social work and to enforce standards in social work practice (Guy, 1994). However, these glimpses of internal discord become immaterial in the face of an extensive body of literature which refutes the ability of nursing, social work and other semi-professions ever to achieve professional status (see, for example, Etzioni, 1969; Salvage, 1988; Llewellyn, 1998). Implicit in these judgements is a perception that both social work and nursing have failed to control their spheres of work. The reasons why the forms of accountability surrounding nursing and social work are different from those in medicine can be found in the inability of the former groups to achieve professional status and its associated rewards.

A number of explanations have been offered for the failure of both nursing and social work to achieve full professional status (see, for example,

Johnson, 1972; Parry and Parry, 1979; Stacey, 1988; Witz, 1992). Of particular interest is Abbott's (1995) view that the public associates social work with altruism rather than science. The same can be said of nursing, but medicine's professional status was based on its originally dubious claim to be scientific as well as altruistic. Medicine's status enabled it to control not only the organisation of nursing work and police its regulation, but also social work. The medical profession's authority over nursing and social work was legitimised by the hegemony of the medical model of practice (and doctors' role as 'guardians' of that knowledge). Clinicians' ability to organise the work of nurses and social workers also derived from their position of authority within state bureaucracies (the local authorities and, after 1948, the NHS). As 'bureau-professionals' (Parry and Parry, 1979) social workers cannot escape the control of an employing organisation (May and Buck, 1998). This state of affairs also applies to nursing. For both occupations, allegiance to the organisation and obedience to bureaucratic modes of accountability have challenged professional discretion and autonomy. Doctors in the NHS may work within bureaucracies but medicine had the advantage of prior establishment of its professional status (and occupational control over nursing and paramedical occupations) before the creation of the NHS. Even so, while this holds as a general tenet, it is important to recognise that the NHS is not an homogenous organisation. In recent history certain areas of the health service have proved more successful in controlling medical practice than others. Paradoxically, the professionalising ambitions of social work were awakened by the emergence of unified SSDs after 1974 (Hugman, 1991). These organisations were based on the Fabian ideal of a combination of professional expertise and "… the regulatory principles of rational administration as the means of accomplishing social welfare" (Newman and Clarke, 1994, p 22). The principle of managerial accountability (Day and Klein, 1987), although not fully developed, was arguably inherent in the ordering of social work at the outset of its professionalising project.

The convenience of history is not by itself a convincing explanation of the preferencing, within medicine, of professional accountability over bureaucratic or managerial forms. The ability of professions to resist bureaucratic (or managerial) regulation is dependent not only on the extent of expert knowledge they claim to use, but also on society's perception of its value (Jamous and Peloille, 1970). Neither nursing, being subordinated to medicine, nor social work could claim such kudos. The mystique of certain forms of knowledge, as well as rebuffing management scrutiny, also secures additional status and protects against popular criticism. The ability of an occupation to sustain its characterisation as altruistic and/or scientific to a public audience is important, given the growing political salience of the appraisal of professional performance within consumerist approaches. With an increasingly alert media and better-informed public this ability may be in decline.

Central to the notion of expert knowledge is the importance of synthesis – the creativity demonstrated by the true professional that is resistant to codification. Jamous and Peloille (1970) capture this idea in the notion of the 'ratio of indeterminacy to technicality'. Put another way, there is a gap between knowledge and its application wherein the professional's interpretive abilities are employed (see Chapter Three). Despite reconfigurations of the nursing role (celebrating the primary nurse and 'bedside practitioner') away from task-oriented functions, hospital nursing is vulnerable to routinisation. Health visiting arguably is less so and may thus be able to claim greater professional creativity (and autonomy), with the resulting ability to resist managerial accountability. However, this assumption has to be tested against two countervailing premises: (a) that the NHS and SSDs are increasingly more managed, with greater levels of accountability exacted from all professional groups involved and (b) that in the specific case of child protection, with its high political sensitivity, the state regulates all professionals more closely through judicial or bureaucratic (rules) processes.

Arguably, in contrast to medicine, the work of social workers and nurses – the 'caring professions'– is undervalued and seen as essentially non-technical and only a little more complicated than women's work in the home. When things go wrong, as evidenced in the findings of numerous public inquiries into child abuse cases, there is little public understanding of the complexity of the social worker's tasks in risk assessment. However, there is a danger in overstating this comparison. Although it is too early to predict the impact on public confidence of recent inquiries into medical activities, it is unlikely that the perceived complexity of clinical work will prevent some loss of the profession's credibility. That the state's acquiescence in the self-regulation of the medical profession may be weakening is evidenced by the new and more robust standards for medical regulation contained in *The NHS Plan* (DoH, 2000a).

Before leaving this discussion of professionalisation, it is important to acknowledge the role of professional cultures in determining susceptibility to different forms of accountability. This not only relates to the significance of values in defining the view that 'street-level' workers (Lipsky, 1980), as opposed to the professions' leaderships, have of professional practice and accountability, but also the importance of those values in accepting alternative modes of accountability. Walby and Greenwell's (1994) account of professional boundaries between doctors and nurses in a hospital setting provides an interesting insight:

> What was striking was that the concept of being a professional for a doctor was such a different notion in practice to what a nurse meant by being a professional.... To many nurses a professional is someone accountable for their practice, guided by rules, and monitored by a senior professional. Rules are annoying at times, but protect nurses from legal challenge and provide security when work involves many stressful situations. To a doctor, a professional is someone who will take responsibility for his/her own judgements and actions, so detailed rules can appear as unprofessional restrictions. (1994, p 52)

These views are the product of the collective experience of two occupational groups over time. Given their profession's history, it is unsurprising that the nurses in Walby and Greenwell's study should offer these views. It helps to explain why professional self-regulation and clinical autonomy in nursing may not be so readily defended against the advancing framework of managerial accountability in the NHS.

Democratic accountability

Democratic accountability in the NHS as a public service is primarily to the Secretary of State for Health, to Parliament and thence to the electorate. Within the NHS, chairs of health authorities and more recently primary care trusts (PCTs) are appointed rather than elected and their boards are accountable to the Secretary of State for their actions. This attenuated, linear model of democratic accountability displaced the alternative proposal for local government control of health services which had been opposed by the BMA "... in both principle and detail" (Carrier and Kendall, 1998, p 65). Thus with the establishment of the NHS, local authorities surrendered their responsibilities for municipal hospitals and the opportunity for the local political accountability of health services was lost. Although local authority members served on the pre-1991 health authorities, they were present as nominees and not elected representatives. However, it is perhaps too simple to attribute this outcome solely to the opposition of the medical profession, important though this was. In the heady idealism of the post-war state, the view prevailed that health care was beyond politics and the prosecution of the NHS' responsibilities could largely be left to the stewardship of health professionals with perhaps an occasional steer from the centre. If, as Klein (1989) suggests, localism was built into the structure of the NHS, it was a localism defined by professional influence rather than representative democracy and with correspondingly weak arrangements for accountability.

Local authorities, in contrast, have not been monopolised by professional élites. County council and unitary authority members are accountable to their electorate for the successful delivery of services, including personal social services, and accordingly exercise authority over the officers (in this case directors of SSDs). Democratic accountability to the local electorate is accompanied by the central line of accountability through the Secretary of State to Parliament. The convention of ministerial accountability to Parliament is an increasingly vulnerable mechanism, however, as a consequence not only of the growing complexity of government but also of the increased dominance of the Cabinet. Additionally, concern has been voiced over the growth of non-elected 'intermediary' organisations responsible for the interpretation of government policy (Rhodes, 1988; Stewart, 1992; see Chapter One of this book). Following the Conservative Party's election in 1979, local authorities lost a number of responsibilities to agencies with limited mechanisms for accountability (Hudson, 1998). The personal social services, however, were not among them; local authorities remain accountable for these services to the Secretary of State and to their local electorates.

The NHS is somewhat less straightforward. The 'hollowing out' of the state thesis is less readily applied to the NHS in that its structure was premised on a degree of devolution, the extent of which has varied over time and according to political disposition. The consensus view is that in recent years the rhetoric of devolution has been confounded by increased regulation (Paton, 1992; Klein, 1995; Powell, 1999) and that the line of accountability between the Secretary of State and the local NHS has survived changes in the wider state. However, the discourse of devolved decision making has allowed the centre to deflect criticism. A good example is the Wessex Regional Health Authority's information technology plan that resulted in a loss of millions of pounds. The regional NHS Management Executive (a classic intermediate body) defended itself, and by default the government, from criticism by the Public Accounts

Committee, by arguing that the responsibility lay with the local health authority (Doig, 1995).

Political accountability in the NHS is therefore intermittently enforceable via the ballot box, but being held to account in this manner is insufficient. Stewart (1995) draws attention to the need to give account and also to listen to what is said. In the NHS, the giving of an account has been compromised by the inadequacy of the questions, which in the past have been preoccupied with inputs and outputs rather than outcomes, and by a (contradictory) allegiance to the principle of professional self-regulation. It has also been weakened by the impoverished culture of public consultation. As Coote and Hunter (1996) argue: "... [accountability] requires a continuing dialogue with the electorate in which the public can both obtain and provide views and information, while the authority is open to scrutiny, listens and responds" (p 79).

The 'continuing dialogue' has, for much of the NHS and its history, been sporadic and limited. The most sustained attempt to establish dialogue, though not entirely successful, was the creation in 1974 of the Community Health Councils (CHCs). The Conservatives' later attempts to strengthen public accountability were mainly conceptualised through consumerist approaches, although choices in the internal market were expressed by purchasers rather than patients (Lupton et al, 1998). These were poor substitutes for the diminished democratic accountability resulting from the removal of local authority representation and the speaking rights of the CHCs on health authorities. For the first time, however, in *Local voices* (NHSME, 1992), health authorities were instructed to consult with local communities over service planning. *The new NHS* (NHS Executive, 1998) and more recently *The NHS Plan* (DoH, 2000a) have described new arrangements for democratic accountability. Signalling the demise of the CHCs, major changes in local services in future are to be assessed by scrutiny committees of local authorities meeting in public. Health authorities will be required to establish advisory forums with a lay membership selected from the local community, to provide a sounding board for determining health priorities and policies. Collectively, the proposals appear to represent a fairly extensive programme of reform which, if effective, should provide greater opportunities for the involvement of the public in key decisions about local services and enhance the accountability of managers and clinicians to their communities.

The development of primary care groups/trusts (PCGs/PCTs) may also increase the possibility of greater local accountability. For the present, however, PCGs remain accountable to health authorities and PCT chairs to the Secretary of State, not to the local electorate. In contrast SSDs, as the responsibility of local authorities, are more open to local public scrutiny and members can be held to account in local elections. Even so, low turnouts at elections and the difficulty of sustaining interest other than in single-issue politics, may be seen to limit the impact of local democracy. In respect of health care, moreover, there is a common presumption that debates are too complex for public consumption. Such conclusions, however, ignore an important principle of community participation: that it may make sense for voters not to concern themselves with issues on which they are unlikely ever to be consulted. The reverse may also be true. If people are regularly consulted about their health care, they may be more inclined to engage with the issues. Ultimately, however, the potency of accountability mechanisms is dependent on organisational and professional cultures.

Managerial accountability

Managerial accountability provides the link between democratic and professional forms. Central to any discussion of accountability is the notion, not only of its indivisibility (that someone can be identified as responsible for certain duties), but that the extent and nature of the duty is clear to both parties – the person held accountable and the person who holds him/her to account. In the NHS and local authority SSDs, the detailed specification of performance objectives may appear to be concerned with the management and direction of the service as a whole. They could accordingly be considered the primary responsibility of service managers, were it not that they require the acquiescence of the key professions. Medical practitioners, nurses and social workers are, in effect, the front-line executors of policies and their clinical decisions have important resource and managerial consequences (and vice versa). Thus the compliance of the key professions with the broadest of aims (to be economic and efficient with resources) is essential to the fulfilment of organisational goals.

Inevitably though, concerns about the effectiveness of professional interventions, be they case working in child protection or the management of illness, have increased interest in more detailed surveillance of professional performance. At its most mundane level, the rationale for this is economic: the wastefulness to the state of uneven performance. Given increased public concern over unacceptable professional performance, however, as demonstrated by successive public inquiries into child abuse over the 1970s and 1980s (DoH, 1991), the state has increasingly intervened to prescribe practice and to clarify the responsibilities of those involved. Similar levels of public concern surround the apparent failure of doctors to provide informed consent and/or to treat patients adequately. More careful elaboration of required standards is likely to follow, and the extent to which the state continues to delegate responsibility for surveillance to the medical profession remains open to renegotiation.

The Griffiths Report on NHS management (DHSS, 1983) (see also Chapter Five) produced a hierarchy of managers who performed to carefully specified individual targets, which were in turn derived from the negotiated agreements between regional health authorities and the Secretary of State, and subsequently between regional health authorities and the NHS Executive. As such it represented a distinct change from the traditional, bureaucratic order and laid the foundation (it was hoped) for more incisive forms of managerial accountability. It was, however, the creation of internal markets that forced reluctant hospital clinicians to engage with trust and NHS goals. Although GP fundholders voluntarily took up their role in the internal market, their participation also required an acceptance of NHS management goals and priorities and conformity with certain procedural standards. It is worth noting that the internal market did not affect the managerial independence of non-fundholders, many of whom were opposed to fundholding on moral (inequity) or practical (additional work) grounds (Robinson and Hayter, 1992).

In contrast, PCGs require the involvement of all practices and therefore afford greater opportunity for managerial accountability. While the duties of PCG boards and their accountability to health authorities are framed by annual agreements, less certainty surrounds the wider 'corporate responsibility' of individual practices. This appears to have been managed by a blend of representation, the unspoken political agreement between profession and state emanating from the significant presence of GPs on PCG boards, by financial incentives encouraging efficient use of secondary services, and by a better defined regime of clinical governance. The more robust arrangements announced in *The NHS Plan* (DoH, 2000a) echo the broader modernisation agenda of government. In the NHS the process is to be steered by the Modernisation Agency which will apply a new Performance Assessment Framework (PAF) to trusts, including PCTs. Trusts and health authorities will earn their autonomy by demonstrating their performance against key targets within the PAF. This new and essentially centralising agenda is not restricted to the NHS. As Chapter

Six describes, *Modernising social services* (DoH, 1998a) also establishes a more elaborate framework for the assessment of SSDs in England, involving locally determined objectives, a performance assessment framework and performance reviews. In combination these should deliver more robust mechanisms for ensuring accountability for child protection services by both agencies. The difficulty for the NHS, however, lies in making GPs accountable for their contribution.

General practice has proved to be a formidable bastion but the managerial foray began with the imposition of the new GP contract in 1990. This made GPs accountable for the provision of certain services to a specified standard, although the penalties were largely financial. While some potential for enhancing consumer power and a form of attenuated accountability lurked in the combination of increased capitation fees and easier exit for dissatisfied patients, in reality this proved a rather ineffectual arrangement (Moon and North, 2000). Nevertheless, the GP contract gave the previously toothless FHSAs, which managed primary care services[2] something to bite with and established the idea that the state could indeed renegotiate the basis on which general medical services were provided. Yet although the manner in which the contract was applied – in the face of robust opposition from the profession – was bold, its content was far from radical. The introduction of Personal Medical Services (PMS) contracts in 1998 provoked less controversy but offered greater potential for the managerial accountability of GPs, since they linked payment for services with performance against specific targets for local needs.

The independence previously enjoyed by GPs will thus in future be reserved to those areas beyond the capacity or inclination of the state to measure. However, this may include the GP role in child protection. Here the guidance to medical practitioners emerging from *Working together* and its subsequent addenda[3] has been somewhat diffident in its approach (see DoH and Welsh Office, 1995 and DoH, 1996). In contrast, the parallel guidance to health visitors details nine responsibilities which include the requirement to "... ensure effective liaison between her staff and those of other agencies" (DoH and Welsh Office, 1995, p 4). The altogether more deferential posture towards the contribution of GPs in child protection processes is consistent with arrangements in the NHS, which have until now deferred to the self-regulatory arrangements of the profession. This position may no longer be tenable.

Conclusion

Those employed by the state who, in effect, allocate scarce resources should be held to account. This was indeed Mill's primary concern – the stewardship of the state's wealth (Mill, 1993). A plausible conclusion would be that systems of managerial accountability have become more sophisticated and more challenging. New public management (NPM), for all the opposition it aroused within the professions, has begun to clarify who is accountable for what. Inevitably the clinical as well as managerial performance of medical practitioners will be assessed as managerial systems of accountability increasingly fuse with professional and democratic forms. Unused to the popular democratic accountability familiar to local authorities, improved consultation between PCGs, PCTs and local communities should encourage both the giving of an account and the dialogue necessary for greater transparency in health service commissioning. If, however, these sentiments are somewhat equivocal in their expression, it is because they recognise the fragility of democratic accountability in the NHS and the intrinsic weakness of the community when confronted by the interests of the state or professions.

Thus, what we see since the mid-1980s is a stealthy usurpation of the dominant mode of accountability in the NHS – professional accountability – by managerial accountability. Its effects have possibly been more potent in the NHS than in local authorities. The latter have also experienced a managerial transformation but have had to attend to local opinion and their electorates, a tension which may mediate the centralising influence of the modernisation plan for the personal social services (DoH, 1998a). The impact of NPM and managerial accountability, however, has not been visited equally on all parts of the NHS or across all professional groups. Nurses, health visitors and social workers, as bureau-professionals have succumbed more easily to increasingly incisive managerial scrutiny. In contrast, the medical profession, the prime target for NPM, has presented more of a challenge and progress has been uneven. Arguably general practitioners, in their business and clinical 'enclaves' (Day and Klein, 1997) have been more able to resist the managerial gaze. Until recently the profession has declined to be publicly accountable for either the husbandry of resources or for clinical standards, a position which neither nursing nor social work could hope (or possibly wish) to sustain.

Applying Benson's theory to child protection, the operation of different professional groups, and to an extent the agencies behind them, reflects substantial inequalities in terms of 'sub-structural' elements such as the level of resources, the dominance of organisational paradigms and the legitimacy of their activities. These inconsistencies both within and between professional groups and between agencies have important consequences for the operationalisation of child protection policies both at the local strategic level (ACPCs) and front-line practice. The following chapter, which traces the multidimensional and shifting dynamics of power between the central and local levels of the NHS, the state and the professions, and between different local interests in health and social care, will further elucidate the wider 'political economy' of child protection.

Notes

[1] Transparency relates to the availability of information that is clear, capable of interpretation and testable against recognisable standards; the condition of indivisibility requires that the locus of accountability ultimately resides in an individual; the power to hold someone to account extends beyond the right to hold someone to account, to having the ability in terms of material and personal resources to do so.

[2] FHSAs also managed dentistry, opthalmic and community pharmacy services, but not community nursing services. Their functions were merged with district health authorities in 1996.

[3] For example, *Child protection: Clarification of arrangements between the NHS and other agencies* (DoH, 1995b); *Child protection: Medical responsibilities* (DoH, 1996); and *Child protection: Guidance for senior nurses, health visitors and midwives* (DoH, 1992b).

FIVE

Power and politics in the NHS

Introduction

Before examining the role of NHS managers and professionals in child protection networks, it is important to gain an understanding of the evolving politics of the NHS. As a near monopoly provider of health care in the UK, the NHS is the principal, though not the sole, 'field of action' for the health policy network. In this network, according to Wistow (1992), the medical profession has played a significant and enduring role. However, the stability of the policy community has been subject to challenge in recent years as Conservative and then Labour governments have attempted to gain greater control over the direction of NHS policies and in doing so have redefined relationships between the state and the professions. As the Benson model indicates (1975, 1983), this shift in external power relations has affected the balance of power within the policy community as well as relationships between elements within the medical profession.

In addition, the devolution of service planning to the local level increases the potential for a more plural process and raises the prospect of local issue networks. In Benson's terms, these may involve the participation of both 'demand' or 'support' groups. The greater number of constituencies to be served may encourage more overt forms of political activity, including between professional interests, as they 'jostle' for position. This chapter will explore these changes in so far as they may impact ultimately on the operationalisation of child protection policies. It will also examine the governability of the NHS and, in association with this, the changing relationship between the state and the professions. The ability of governments to implement health policy will be discussed in relation to changing centre–local relations and, in particular, the compliance of key professional groups. The role of the health professions will be explored, as will the place of the 'silent citizen'[1] in NHS politics. While concluding that the medical profession, and increasingly general practice, still exerts considerable influence within the health policy community, it appears that the state has succeeded in exerting greater control over the profession as a whole. The state–medical profession dynamic is, however, only one consideration in local provider networks. The interagency and interprofessional politics within networks are contextualised by the firm regulatory steer of the centre.

Governing the NHS: ambiguity and inertia

If a necessary precondition to government is purpose, then the difficulties encountered in governing the NHS are in part attributable to the impossibility of its mission. The grandiose objectives of the service – to provide equal access for equal need to health care free at the point of use – have been beset by ambiguities. The difficulty of the task has been exacerbated by what, for Klein (1989), is a fundamental tension within the NHS: the centre's need to control in order to satisfy national accountability and the recognition that the NHS should not be maintained without local autonomy.

Thus, while the idea of local autonomy fortuitously combined pragmatic necessity with political expediency, it was a *modus operandi* that, in the first three decades of the NHS, subverted the policy initiatives of the centre. When there was sufficient will to challenge the status quo, considerable political energy was required to overturn institutionalised inertia and, in some quarters, intransigence. The huge and complex organisation that was created in 1948 was, for Eckstein (1958), an outcome of administrative rationality. By abandoning earlier proposals to give control to local authorities, however, the opportunities for integrated and accountable local services were lost. What emerged, the tripartite structure and its associated administrative arrangements, represented important concessions to the various interests involved (Willcocks, 1967; Carrier and Kendall, 1998) including those of an heterogeneous medical profession. A fragmented structure resulted, which was difficult to administer and which marginalised community/public health and primary care elements. Both health visiting and general practice were situated in the administrative hinterland. Community nursing was under the control of local health authorities and GPs, who retained their independent contractor status and were distantly administered to by Executive Councils.

The medical profession was comprehensively represented at the Ministry of Health, where there were both professional and administrative hierarchies (Ham, 1999), as well as at every level of the NHS. Overt displays of medical power were seldom required, as doctors exerted influence through their role as service providers and through the deference accorded to medical opinion (Haywood and Alaszewski, 1980; Ham, 1981). As Eckstein graphically reported:"At all the hospital committees I attended, I did not hear a professional opinion overturned" (1958, p 230). The likelihood of opposition, or at least robust debate, from either appointed lay members or administrators within the service was limited (Hunter, 1980; Ham, 1981). Non-decision making – the mobilisation of bias which restricts decision making to non-contestable issues (Bachrach and Baratz, 1970) in favour of the status quo of powerful medical interests – was also evident in relationships between Whitehall and the regional boards (Klein, 1989). In addition, the medical profession was able to muster formidable political force at the heart of policy making. Thus Webster observes that the BMA possessed: "... an unenviable record for assaults against the government of the day on matters great and small" (1998, p 45).

Medicine was by far the most powerful interest within NHS politics and due deference was accorded to it by politicians, administrators and by the numerically significant nursing profession. Hospital nursing, as noted earlier, was administratively separate from district nursing and health visiting, which were the responsibility of local authorities until the 1974 reorganisation of the NHS. Community nursing services were controlled by medical officers of health: doctors who had little status in the medical hierarchy but who, until 1974, were "... firmly in charge of (their) empire" (Owens and Glennerster, 1990, p 8). The picture was a little more complicated within the NHS where nursing had some control over the local organisation of its labour. Nursing's influence was further enhanced by the Salmon Report (Ministry of Health, 1966), which created a managerial hierarchy for nursing, and by the consensus management teams (consisting of doctors, nurses and administrators) introduced in the 1974 reorganisation. The arrangement required that nurses on the management team were consulted before any major change was made and, as a result: "... could largely expect their views to be heeded" (Clay, 1989, p 116). Despite this, nursing influence remained largely conspicuous by its absence (Hunter, 1980; Haywood and Alaszewski, 1980; Ham, 1981). The profession's opinions carried weight in nursing matters but were unlikely to deviate from the received (medical) view in other discussions. At the national level, nursing's contribution to mainstream debates about the health service was inaudible. Nursing was seen, and regarded itself, to be inconsequential to these debates (Clay, 1989) and generally did not consider political activity to be consonant with a vocational calling.

If the early structures of the NHS were fashioned to provide professional groups and particularly the medical profession with an influential role in decision making, little such opportunity was extended to the citizen or to patient groups. The organisation of the NHS during the 1950s, 1960s and 1970s reflected a belief that professional, and particularly medical, opinion should lead local decisions and contribute to national policy making. This paternalistic approach was reflected in the constituency of the stable policy community in the health sector (Wistow, 1992) from which patient groups were excluded. Administrative tidiness and the appeasement of medical interests were deemed preferable to local accountability. The layperson's voice in NHS decision making was required to be informed and rational rather than political and partisan and this limited opportunities for democratic representation. The 1974 reorganisation excluded lay members from consensus management but, after protests from the Labour opposition, the constitution of area health authorities (AHAs) was changed in 1975 so that a third of members were selected from local government. In addition, Community Health Councils (CHCs) – which most closely fit Benson's description of localised 'support groups' – were established with the dual remit of representing the views of the public to the newly created district management teams and advising the public on the process of making a complaint. Community Health Councils made themselves enough of a nuisance to invoke the dissatisfaction of government, but underfunding weakened their efforts (Moon and Lupton, 1995). Thus in the early years of the NHS there was little formal opportunity for citizen participation within the NHS and nothing – until the creation of the Association of Community Health Councils, England and Wales – representing lay opinion within the wider policy community[1].

Challenging the interests

A combination of circumstances propelled the NHS towards the watershed changes that followed the NHS management inquiry (DHSS, 1983). The Conservatives' victory in 1979 elected a government that did not share in the social democratic welfare consensus and which had learned important lessons from the experiences of the previous Labour government. One of its first actions was to implement a recommendation of the Royal Commission on the NHS (1979) to abolish the AHAs. This excised a tier of bureaucracy but, since AHAs were coterminous with local authorities and had up to one third local authority membership, their disappearance also impaired the coordination of local health and social care services. For the Conservatives, however, the difficulties of the NHS went deeper than that of unnecessary administrative layers. They gradually etched a model of health care which, while committed to controlling expenditure and remedying inefficiencies, also theoretically supported the notion of consumer choice, a more competitive professional environment and the active management of health care (Salter, 1998).

The 1983 Griffiths Report reforms ushered in a cadre of NHS managers more attentive to the requirements of policy makers (DHSS, 1983). Doctors were encouraged to participate as managers in an effort to synthesise clinical and resource management, but the response was generally poor and the impact of new public management (NPM) on the NHS during the first few years was weak (Harrison et al, 1989; Strong and Robinson, 1990). In contrast, the Griffiths Report had a significant effect on nursing, which opposed the proposals but failed to mobilise support from an uninterested public. Losing its traditional professional hierarchies, nursing experienced a loss of power and value within the NHS.

However there were other, less immediately discernible effects. Strong and Robinson (1990) argue that the Griffiths Report reforms broke the power sharing agreement between Whitehall and the professions that had traditionally characterised the health policy community. The medical profession in particular had been found wanting in its stewardship of the NHS. More fundamentally, managerialism began to effect a change in the discourse of health care, emphasising the need for resource management rather than the primacy of individual patient needs. In doing so it subverted the traditional claim of the medical profession to know what is best for the patient and the associated justification of its control over resource decisions. Challenged by hospital consultants, however, managers lacked the necessary disciplinary levers to force decisions through and change remained incremental and dependent on negotiation (Strong and Robinson, 1990).

If the medical profession had been able to defy the Griffiths Report reforms, the creation of the purchaser/provider split was another matter. The review which preceded the White Paper, *Working for patients* (DoH, 1989a), excluded traditional members of the policy community and fractured entrenched procedural rules of the game (Wistow, 1992). Although the newly named family health services authorities (FHSAs) remained separate from district health authorities (DHAs) there was a clear chain of command between them and the NHS Management

Executive. Their previous independence, despite recommendations by the Royal Commission (1979) that they be assimilated in health authorities, was in part attributable to the entrenched opposition of the BMA and other medical interest groups, who feared a dilution of their power. District health authorities were in theory given the freedom to commission local health services; in practice their operational discretion was circumscribed by the welter of Whitehall directives. Subject to performance goals, enforced by rewards and sanctions (Paton, 1992; Klein, 1995), the DHAs operated on the basis of "freedom within boundaries" (Hoggett, 1991, p 251).

The new, more functional structure signalled that the government meant business. The internal market reforms were introduced despite the opposition of the medical profession. Clinicians now had to adopt different strategies and work closely with managers to secure contracts, their historic influences over the development of health care displaced to purchasers, including GPs. Fundholding represented an incorporation into management by stealth. Although GP fundholders enjoyed a new-found influence in the NHS, they were committed to managing resources. As fundholders were enlisted by health authorities to serve on strategic commissioning bodies, they became corporately responsible for the interpretation of national priorities and initiatives. Locality commissioning groups involving both GP fundholders and GPs were similarly placed. The quid pro quo for increased prestige and influence was exposure to mainstream NHS management cultures. A more forthright challenge to the traditional autonomy of GPs, however, materialised in the form of a new contract, which defined the GP's role with more precision and created targets linked to differential payments. The underlying rationale was to reward behaviour that would encourage retention of patients, improve immunisation and screening rates and encourage health promotion. Despite an outcry over the original, non-negotiated contract, GPs responded to what were essentially management-defined standards and targets with enthusiasm. The GP contract played to the acquisitive nature of GPs and political sensitivities were forgotten in the pursuit of targets.

Whereas control over the medical profession was considerably strengthened by the purchaser–provider split and the GP contract, the effect on nursing was less dramatic, precisely because nursing was already assimilated within NHS management. That is not to say, however, that the introduction of contracts did not bring with it subtle changes in the power relationships between GPs and community nursing. Since the early 1970s, both district nurses and health visitors had been attached to

GP practices but, unlike practice nurses, were not employed by GPs. With the development of internal markets, GP fundholders became the customers of community nursing services. They were able to specify contracts for a range of district nurse and health visiting services, including child health surveillance. This altered the dynamics of GP–community nurse relationships (Hiscock and Pearson, 1995), reinforcing historic imbalances of status between primary health care team members, and supplanting health visiting's traditional preventative role with a medicalised and commercialised model of service provision (Symonds, 1997).

The Conservatives' reforms did little to encourage democracy in the NHS, though their performance was no worse than that of previous governments. Essentially the internal market reforms promoted the idea of patients as consumers, who could express their will through choice rather than voice. Such choices in relation to hospital treatment and general practice were largely illusory, leading to the conclusion that the internal market was intended more as a strategy to manipulate medical performance according to the requirements of resource management. Another initiative with an apparent democratic purpose enjoined health authorities and subsequently locality commissioning groups to consult with local communities over service development (NHSME, 1992). However, Lupton et al (1998) suggest that the extent to which consultative processes engaged with the health care planning process was uneven. In local policy making, as with health service policy development at the national level, the influence of the citizen (Benson's demand group) or even of service user interest groups (Benson's support groups), has been tentative.

The third way: redefining the rules?

> The reality is that a million patients every day rely on the skills and judgement of highly trained frontline professionals, so the NHS cannot be run from Whitehall. (DoH, 2000a)

The New Labour government sought to develop a 'third way' between the social democratic welfarism of old Labour and the neo-liberalism that characterised Thatcherism. This was an essentially pragmatic approach, supporting a mixed economy of welfare but rejecting the market fundamentalism of the new Right. While encouraging accountability, open government, active citizenship and equal access, the project also stressed the responsibility of individuals. Despite the quote above, the third way did not imply any relinquishing of control by the centre. Powell (1999, p 364) detects formidable disciplinary arrangements and concludes that, in spite of Labour's intention to eschew systems of 'command and control,"... it is possible that there may be effective command and control for the first time" (p 364).

This extension of central control has been an evolutionary process starting at the top. The government's modernisation plan amounts to a comprehensive strategy for securing greater control over the periphery by surveillance and a system of rewards or penalties. A chief executive with responsibility for the NHS, public health and social services will be accountable to a newly created Modernisation Board for the delivery of the proposed *NHS Plan* (DoH, 2000a). For all its glowing endorsements ("Our family doctors are a real source of strength for the NHS";"Hospital doctors do a brilliant job" – DoH, 2000a, sections 8.2 and 8.12), the *NHS Plan* indicates a much more robust approach to health professionals that contrasts with the tone of earlier initiatives. The White Papers[2] published in December 1997 and January 1998, eschewed the internal market and the alleged competitive environment in favour of a more collaborative approach. General practitioners retained considerable commissioning power in local service development in England, but decision making in the primary care groups (PCGs) was to be broadened to include community nursing and representation from social services (see Chapter Six for discussion in relation to collaboration between the NHS and SSDs). Even where PCGs evolved to primary care trusts (PCTs), independent organisations with comprehensive commissioning responsibilities, key positions on the executive committees were to be held by professionals.

The strategy of "centrally controlled devolution" (Light, 1998, p 431) was further developed by *The NHS Plan* (DoH, 2000a). Despite the rhetoric of 'earned autonomy', which PCTs can secure for good behaviour, the plan sets out a cat's cradle of measures designed to mould the performance of purchasers and providers according to policy requirements. Overall, however, the political influence of the medical profession and, to a lesser degree, that of other professional groups involved in the PCGs/ PCTs, may be only slightly compromised. In place of consensus management of the 1970s, consensual agreements are now to be reached in local commissioning, the difference being that GPs, rather than hospital clinicians, are afforded the greatest influence in resource allocation. The nursing profession's hopes of acquiring much greater local and, therefore, national influence, not illogically fuelled by the egalitarian tone of the

The new NHS (DoH, 1997), were dashed as a consequence of some determined lobbying by the BMA in the lead-up to PCGs. This secured both the position of chair and the majority membership of GPs on PCG boards. Control of the PCGs was deemed of critical importance, as was the need to protect the independent contractor status of the profession (Chisholm, 1998a). The reason for this anxiety becomes apparent in the budgetary arrangements for PCGs that for the first time included GP prescribing and practice infrastructure costs as well as allocations for hospital and community health services. As a consequence, all GPs were locked into a system that required resource management of general practice as well as community and hospital services, although significantly this did not include general medical services (payments for the doctors' services).

As well as imposing budgetary discipline on primary care, PCGs/PCTs may provide the medium by which GPs are exposed to different values and knowledge systems. Above all, while allowing local professionals discretion in the commissioning choices they make, thereby utilising professional knowledge and experience of local services, PCGs/PCTs also constitute the means whereby one of the most autonomous branches of medicine may be persuaded or obliged to conform to national requirements. The quid pro quo is that they have acquired great influence in local health service planning. Equally, it is possible to surmise the impact that community nursing and health visiting may have on service developments from their positions on PCGs and, perhaps more importantly, PCTs. Although the imbalance in numbers between community nurses and GPs will not encourage an influential voice, health visiting may be able to operate with greater effect from its position within PCTs, whose longevity should also encourage a greater political sophistication in local health visiting. This may be important in the development of local child services and in child protection work as will, no doubt, the presence of social services representatives.

In the health policy community and at local level, lay participation has made little tangible impact on policy decisions. Labour's declared objective was to increase both individual (patient) and collective (citizen) voice in service evaluation and planning (DoH, 1998a). Initially, the responsibility for so doing was placed with health authorities who, with local authorities, were responsible for the development of the local health improvement programmes (HImPs). Recognising the need to restore public confidence in the NHS, the Labour government stressed the importance of PCGs and PCTs working with local communities to develop greater local ownership of services. However, the history of public involvement in general practice and primary care commissioning is not convincing (Agass et al, 1991; Myles et al, 1998; Moon and North, 2000). A study of public involvement in PCGs in London found a degree of uncertainty about how to promote involvement, with the majority perceiving that that lay members had the primary responsibility for this aspect of their work. Although there was acceptance of the principle, public involvement was not given a high priority (DoH, 2000a). This may be about to change as the *NHS Plan* proposes extensive arrangements for public representation on NHS monitoring agencies, on the professions' regulatory bodies and on health authority advisory forums. In addition, all-party 'scrutiny committees' of local authorities will have the power to refer major planned changes in local services to a new national Independent Reconfiguration Panel, which will have one third lay membership. While these initiatives may not affect the working of PCGs directly, they do signify a changed approach to public participation in the governance of the NHS.

Conclusion

If, at the inception of the NHS, there was a degree of political naivety, this quickly faded. The assumptions that the service would somehow perform in harmony with the vague ideals associated with it soon evaporated. From the early years the need to reconcile national accountability and local autonomy was evident, but accountability was defined primarily in terms of financial probity. Subsequently the gap between national policies and their implementation at local level became more evident and more problematic against a backdrop of financial stringency. In effect the policy failures of the 1970s signified a divergence from the model of health care which had previously prevailed in corporatist relationships between the state and medical profession. They also demonstrated that the governance of the NHS, even considering the need for local discretion in the implementation of policy, was precarious and relied on a correspondence of values between the centre and periphery that clearly did not obtain.

This scenario does not square well with traditional accounts of policy communities, which require a degree of ideological harmony and reciprocity. In the case of the NHS the medical members within the community's core, the BMA and the Royal Colleges (Klein, 1989), were required to carry the membership on policy, but there are clear examples of policy implementation failures, which subsequently challenged the integrity of the health policy community. The more substantial threat to the policy community came with the Conservative Party's election to office in 1979. The Conservatives not only redefined the terms on which health care was to be provided – constraint, efficiency and effectiveness became the goals rather than the means of improving health care – but rejected the very idea of a health policy community (Wistow, 1992) and with it the idea that implementation of policy required the tacit consent of the medical profession. The Conservatives bypassed the policy community and concentrated instead on engaging the support of fundholding 'street-level' workers (Lipsky, 1980), using the lure of increased influence and financial reward.

To a degree, the medical profession was rehabilitated under the 1997 Labour government. Concessions to the General Medical Services Committee in the lead-up to the establishment of PCGs reflected the need to win the support of the profession at the expense of other stakeholders, including the nursing profession. Pragmatism was evident on both sides; for their part GPs recognised the potential of PCGs and PCTs to threaten their power, income and working relationships with patients (Chisholm, 1998b; North et al, 1999). There are, however, substantial differences between the deal struck in 1948 at the start of the NHS and that bartered between Labour and the General Medical Services Committee in 1998. The 1948 negotiations enrolled GPs in a NHS but at arm's-length from any administrative supervision; the 1998 arrangements co-opted GPs in the planning of local services including, for the first time, GP services. The centre's ability and determination to fashion the broad direction of service development now extends to general practice. Proposals to review the General Medical Services contract and to promote salaried employment for GPs (DoH, 2000a) are likely to herald the most significant changes yet in the management of general practice.

As discussed in Chapter Four, the unique political power of the medical profession was defined through its clinical autonomy and its claim to complex knowledge, capable of being assessed only by peers. That autonomy has been weakened as new initiatives have shifted the criteria for professional performance and increasingly insisted on more pluralistic and independent forms of audit. Reports of the demise of the medical profession are, however, premature. It remains an effective and significant entity in national and local health politics. Discussions in this chapter lead to the conclusion that the medical profession continues to play a central role within the health policy community. Other groups, such as the nursing profession and lay interest groups, remain on the periphery to be consulted on specific issues as before (see Wistow, 1992). There are, however, significant differences. To maintain its place, medicine has had to accept paradigmatic changes in health policy, borne of social and economic necessity. These have elevated the role of preventive medicine and of long-term care, have relocated the 'place' of care to community and have compelled medicine to open itself up to greater scrutiny.

In respect of local child protection provider networks, the implications of these developments are likely to be mixed. In spite of their significance, GPs can elect not to become involved in local child protection networks. Unlike health visiting and social work and the organisations involved, the *resources* (money, authority and legitimisation) to be gained from their involvement are for the present marginal. On the other hand, *Modernising social services* (DoH, 1998a) and *The NHS Plan* (DoH, 2000a) signal a more robust approach to the operations of both SSDs and the NHS 'family' in relation to child protection.

This raises the stakes for both agencies and professions since the fulfilment of programme requirements, adequate funding and public legitimisation (Benson's sub-structural processes) are bound up with the state's more pressing agenda. Unlike other areas of health and social care, however, the distinctive nature of the child protection process makes this a somewhat closed policy area at local as well as national level. Other than in cases of spectacular failure, the performance of those involved will be judged largely by the centre. The extent to which the stronger mandate to cooperate will subdue fragmenting interests is open to question. As the next chapter identifies, the histories of the agencies and of the professional groups involved in child protection suggest that there remains much to do.

Notes

[1] The concept of citizen-as-participant is different from either the demand or support groups identified by Benson, but is deemed more appropriate to a publicly funded service. As Benson (1983) indicates, patient interest groups such as the CHCs could function as either 'demand' or 'support' groups.

[2] There were separate White Papers: for England (*The new NHS: Modern, dependable*, DoH, 1997), Wales (DoH and Welsh Office, 1998, *Putting patients first*), and Scotland (*Designed to care: Renewing the National Health Service in Scotland*, Scottish Office DoH, 1997).

SIX

Reluctant partners:
the experience of health and
social care collaboration

Introduction

> The Government has made it one of its top priorities since coming to
> office to bring down the 'Berlin Wall' that can divide health and social
> services and create a system of integrated care that puts users at the
> centre of service provision. (DoH, 1998a, p 997)

The 'Berlin Wall' seen to divide health and social care services featured
strongly in the policy debates of the late 1990s. Particularly in respect of
community care services, but also in provision for children and their
families, effective service interventions were seen to be frustrated by a
lack of coordination between different professionals, agencies and/or
departments. In the child protection context, successive official inquiries
identified failures in communication or interagency/interprofessional
collaboration as a major contributory factor (DHSS, 1974; London
Borough of Bexley, 1982; London Borough of Brent, 1985; London
Borough of Greenwich, 1987). Earlier chapters have set out some of the
potential barriers to interprofessional and multiagency working, in
particular the difficulties resulting from different, and possibly conflicting,
disciplinary approaches and service paradigms. They have also highlighted
problems arising from the diverse systems of regulation and accountability
surrounding network participants. This chapter examines the impact of
central policy initiatives designed to enhance collaboration between health
and social services authorities and identifies further areas of organisational
resistance to effective joint working in child protection. After providing
a brief history of collaboration between the NHS and social care agencies,
the chapter examines the implications for local provider networks of the
1997 Labour government's modernisation agenda.

A brief history of health and social care collaboration

As we have seen, from its inception the NHS was kept administratively separate from the other two pillars of the welfare state – social care and social security. Effective collaboration between health and social care services was hampered by divisions between and within the NHS and the local authorities. Within the NHS, the core medical services – general practice and hospitals – were located outside local government control, effectively splitting them organisationally from the community or public health services – medical officers of health, community nursing and environmental health – which remained under the local authorities (Honigsbaum, 1989; Ottewill and Wall, 1990; see Chapter Five of this book). Within the local authorities there was duplication and overlap between the administratively separate departments of personal social services, children's services and mental health services. In the face of this fragmentation, subsequent years were marked by successive attempts to forge connections between the NHS and local authorities in areas of shared responsibility.

The 1962 hospital plan (Ministry of Health, 1962), the health and welfare plans of 1963 (Ministry of Health, 1963) and the formation of a new Department of Health and Social Security (DHSS) in 1968 represented early moves in this direction and the reorganisation of both health and local authorities in the early 1970s explicitly aimed to improve the capacity for coordinated action (Wistow, 1982; Booth, 1981; Hallett, 1995). A government working party set up in 1973 attempted to tighten the relationship further. Rather than the occasional cooperation of two agencies which otherwise continued to operate separately, the objective was to stimulate "genuinely collaborative methods of working throughout the process of planning" (DHSS, 1973, quoted in Booth, 1981, p 25). The resulting 1973 NHS Reorganisation Act charged local and health authorities with a statutory duty to establish formal collaborative structures for joint planning and provision of services. These structures included Joint Consultative Committees (JCCs) and joint care planning teams. In order to provide a 'tangible inducement' to collaboration, the provision of joint finance was introduced in 1976 (Booth, 1981, p 27).

Despite these initiatives, and pressure for organisational integration from documents such as *Better services for the mentally handicapped* (DHSS,1971) and *Better services for the mentally ill* (DHSS, 1975), the evidence suggests that interagency collaboration over the 1970s was beset by tensions at both policy and operational levels. Practical obstacles to joint work resulted from differences in management structures, organisational timescales, geographical boundaries and finance systems (Allsop, 1984; Hunter and Wistow, 1987). These were overlaid by problems of 'departmentalism' or 'bureaucratic rivalry' (Stoker, 1991) and professional defensiveness/imperialism (Challis et al, 1988; Hudson, 1992), particularly on the part of the new social care professionals (Hallett, 1995).

Commentators argue that the problem lay with central government's concern with establishing the formal mechanisms for collaboration, such as joint planning and the JCCs, rather than creating the incentives for organisations to work together (Wistow, 1982; Hudson, 1992). Without the latter, the mechanisms themselves were always likely to prove insufficient to the task. The joint finance structure, for example, was largely used to fund small-scale initiatives at the interface of the two agencies (Chapman et al, 1995). At best it served as a form of 'parallel planning' (Hunter and Wistow, 1987, p 13); at worst it degenerated into "a local professional power game" (Glennerster et al, 1983, p 90). Other mechanisms were seen to have performed little better: the JCCs were dismissed as merely 'talking shops' (Butcher, 1995, p 70) and the joint care planning teams were disregarded as 'clumsy and ineffectual' (Challis et al, 1988, p 181). None of this was assisted by a lack of overall direction from the then DHSS (Hudson, 1992) within which there was little organisational or strategic coordination between its three main areas of responsibility: health, social security and the personal social services (Nairne, 1984). The result was little improvement in strategic collaboration or in the coordination of services to individual clients (Hunter and Wistow, 1987).

Despite these failures, the issue of interagency cooperation remained a central policy concern over the 1980s. In the field of community care, a series of official reports (Audit Commission, 1986b; National Audit Office, 1987) continued to stress the need for interagency collaboration. These pressures culminated in the 1988 Griffiths Report which, in proposing a shift in the role of local authorities from direct provision to purchasing, recommended they develop a comprehensive planning system in conjunction with health, housing and agencies in the voluntary and independent sector. The subsequent White Papers *Working for patients* and *Caring for people* (DoH, 1989a, 1989b) and the 1990 NHS and Community Care Act and supplementary policy guidance (DoH, 1990) clarified the different responsibilities of social and health authorities and attempted to encourage a more rational and coordinated approach to the development of services. Local and health authorities would each produce annual plans and ensure they were complementary by agreeing at an early stage the details of "... who does what, for whom, when, at what cost and who pays" (DoH, 1990, paras 2.11/12). Yet again, however, the planning mechanism failed to deliver. As local authorities struggled with the process (Moore, 1992) the majority of plans comprised statements of position rather than strategic objectives (Wistow et al, 1993), ending up as little more than an 'annual paper exercise' (Salter and Salter, 1993).

Part of the problem was the assumption that agencies were generally inclined to cooperate. In the context of the ongoing restructuring of public sector services, however, this may have been naive. In particular it may have underestimated the growing tensions between agencies as a result of different arrangements surrounding resource acquisition and demand management. As Benson argues, a central objective for any organisation is maintaining "... orderly, reliable patterns of resource flow" (Benson, 1975, p 237). As soon as it emerged as the "hidden fourth pillar of the welfare state" (Salter, 1998, p 158), the community care sector grew exponentially. More and more groups of actual or potential service users were added to the original client groups of people with mental illness, older people and people with learning disabilities. The overall level of demand, moreover, was heightened by an emphasis on the 'empowerment' of users and carers and by the creation of the 'quasi-purchaser' role of the social services care manager.

The inability of the national tax base to underwrite the expansion of community care services placed considerable pressure on the state, at both central and local levels, to control demand. This was to be accomplished by the "... two parameters of cash limits and assessments of need" (Select Committee of the House of Commons, 1993, p 42). These two mechanisms, however, impacted differently on health and social care agencies. Whereas rights to social care services are inherently conditional, depending crucially on "... what is available and affordable" (DoH, 1989b, p 20), this is not the case for health care services. Although the right to health care has always been contingent on professional decisions, it has been (historically at least) less overtly subject to explicit resource limitations and has, in the main, remained free at the point of delivery. The very different positions of the NHS and social care agencies in respect of the conditions of the supply/demand for services represents a core tension at the heart of community care services. As health and social services authorities both strove to respond to rising levels of demand, the community care arena was increasingly characterised by disputes over the demarcation of 'social' and 'health' care needs and by 'cost-shunting' between agencies (Hudson, 1997, p 2).

In particular, health authorities were increasingly disinclined to transfer money from their relatively protected budgets for specific community care client groups to what were seen to be the relatively unprotected general community care budgets of local authorities (Salter, 1998). The Griffiths Report on community care (Griffiths, 1988) had recommended the establishment of 'ring-fenced' community care budgets to facilitate the transfer of funds. The government's subsequent failure to implement this recommendation, Salter argues, was not entirely unrelated to the 'unwelcome visibility' it would have experienced when those budgets proved inadequate to meet the rapidly expanding demand for services (1998, p 170). As the Audit Commission acknowledged, organisational collaboration would remain inherently difficult: "... as long as services are funded through discrete routes and controlled by separate bodies with different priorities and accountabilities" (1992, p 35).

Problems with interagency collaboration also resulted from the lack of geographical 'fit' between NHS and social care agencies. Before the DHA and FHSA mergers, only around one quarter of the DHAs and SSDs were coterminous. Others, as the Audit Commission remarked, were "hopelessly entangled" (1992, p 12). This difficulty was not assisted by the introduction of internal markets in both health and social care services nor by further local government reorganisation. There is evidence that the greater fragmentation of the new mixed economy of health and social care, especially within the NHS, hindered effective planning and coordination, not least by increasing the sheer number of agencies/sectors involved (Barker, 1996, p 33; Dobson, 1992). Collaboration was also hampered as contracts focused organisational effort on shorter timescales and a competitive and 'inward looking' culture inhibited the sharing of necessary information (Lewis, 1993; Audit Commission, 1994; Donaldson and Creswell, 1994; Hudson, 1994; Sadlar, 1994; Barker, 1996).

Collaboration in children's services

While the policy attention given to interagency working focused mainly on community care services, there was growing concern over the 1980s about poor cooperation in children's services. This was driven in particular by a series of official inquiries into child abuse, as we discuss below, but was not confined to child protection services. Thus the report of the Health Advisory Service into the provision of services for 'disturbed' adolescents commented on the unwillingness of the agencies to share knowledge and skills. Without better interprofessional cooperation, it argued, "... no comprehensive solutions can be found to the problems posed and faced by these young people" (HAS, 1986, quoted in Blyth and Milner, 1990, p 195). Some attempt was made to address this issue with *Working together* (DHSS and Welsh Office, 1988), but it was not until the 1989 Children Act that the formal requirement for interagency collaboration was made in respect of the provision of children's services.

The need for services from a variety of professions and agencies was strongly emphasised in the Act. The legislation made very clear that the multidimensional nature of children's needs required the involvement of a range of complementary services. In addition to health and social services, these would include local education authorities, housing departments and the voluntary and independent sectors. The explicit intention of the Act was to improve child protection interventions, not merely by better communication between agencies, but by active interagency and interprofessional collaboration at both strategic and operational levels. This would involve the creation of systems in which different professions and agencies could work together to produce joint assessments and provide ongoing care. The focus of the Act, moreover, was not solely on child protection services but on services for children in need more widely. As Tunstill et al argue, the Children Act in this way "... expanded considerably" the traditional interpretation of interagency collaboration (1996, p 42).

Following the evidence of the abuse of children in residential care (the 'Pindown' report, Levy and Kahan, 1991), and the Social Services Inspectorate review of the residential service (Utting, 1991), a circular was issued to local authorities 'advising' them to draw up more coordinated and coherent strategies for the development of all children's services (DoH, 1992a, p 18). This contained the 'expectation' that this would be done in collaboration with other relevant agencies, but was accompanied by no similar circular to health or local education authorities (Sutton, 1995). The 1994 Audit Commission report on the coordination of health and social care services for children, however, noted a continued overlap of provision and a widespread lack of control between the agencies. Its recommendation that the production of children's services plans be made joint and mandatory and should reflect common values and priorities as well as details of joint operational interests was implemented in 1996. But as Sutton (1995) comments, despite increased emphasis on the joint nature of the plans, the official guidance still presented the SSD as the lead agency and was based on the assumption that the priorities of the Children Act would coincide with those of 'other players' such as health and local education authorities.

In the child protection context, pressure for collaboration came from a succession of child abuse inquiries over the 1970s and 1980s. The 1974 report of the Maria Colwell inquiry, in particular, was crucial in determining the pivotal role of the interagency system. The report was clear that the "... greatest and most obvious" failure of the system was "... the lack of, or ineffectiveness of, communication and liaison" (DHSS, 1974, p 86). The Colwell inquiry was central in establishing the formal structures of the interagency child protection process. Area Review Committees (ARCs) were to oversee the development of policy, training and the organisation of joint case work, and a central record or register of child abuse cases was to be established to ensure "... good communication between the many disciplines involved" (DHSS, 1974, p 1). The operation of these registers was further refined in subsequent departmental circulars (DHSS, 1976, 1980). They would now underpin the strategic planning and developmental role of the ARCs – redesignated in 1988 as Area Child Protection Committees (ACPCs) – and inform individual case management. In this way the function of the registers explicitly shifted from that of facilitating communication to that of underpinning collaboration (Gibbons ct al, 1995). The Colwell inquiry also reaffirmed the importance of the multidisciplinary child protection conference, which "lies at the heart of interagency collaboration" (Hallett, 1995, p 166). This mechanism was introduced in 1950 on the recommendation of the Home Office to bring together any relevant statutory or voluntary services in the area to consider the needs of particular children and to agree how best to respond to them (Home Office, 1950).

The message about interagency collaboration was to remain constant through successive child abuse inquiry reports. Thus the Jasmine Beckford inquiry stressed the importance of cooperation between local and health authorities and recommended imposing a formal duty on health authorities to report any concerns to SSDs (London Borough of Brent, 1985). The subsequent investigation into the death of Kimberley Carlile highlighted the 'fudge of divided responsibilities' between the relevant authorities and strongly recommended the creation of a joint organisation incorporating child care and child health services (London Borough of Greenwich, 1987). This was further endorsed by the Cleveland inquiry (Secretary of State for Social Services, 1988), which recommended the establishment of specialist interagency assessment teams, and in the subsequent Rochdale and Orkney cases (DoH and SSI, 1990a, 1990b).

Mandated coordination

Watton (1993) among others (Hallett and Stevenson, 1980; Parton 1985) argues that the dominant view that child protection failures resulted from poor collaboration meant that the policy solution focused on the development of more effective procedures and systems for interagency working. The outcome has been strong central scrutiny and direction of child protection activity. As described in Chapter Two, via a series of guidance documents and circulars, the core policy community has effectively attempted to 'mandate coordination' (Hallett and Birchall, 1992, p 32). As a result, the role of existing interagency mechanisms has shifted from that of facilitating communication to that of underpinning joint working. The first official guidance for *Working together* (DHSS and Welsh Office, 1988) in child protection sought to clarify the roles of various agencies and advised the creation of interagency specialist assessment teams. Subsequent revisions consolidated the emphasis on collaborative work in both process and content. Thus the 1991 version, produced jointly by the Home Office, DoH, Department of Education and Science (DES) and the Welsh Office, recommended that collaboration characterise all stages of an individual 'case career', from referral and investigation through registration planning and eventual deregistration. Further clarification of the arrangements for joint working was provided in a series of addenda covering arrangements between the NHS and other agencies (DoH and Welsh Office, 1995), guidance to doctors working with child protection agencies (DoH, 1996) and guidance for senior nurses, health visitors and midwives and their managers (DoH and Standing Nursing and Midwifery Advisory Committee, 1997).

Despite increased central direction and the establishment of formal structures for interagency collaboration, evidence from DoH-funded research in the mid-1990s revealed that considerable problems remained in child protection. Hallett (1995), for example, found little implementation of the recommendation that collaboration should characterise all stages of an individual case. The situation was just the opposite: "... following the peak of inter-agency involvement at the initial child protection conference, it diminishes thereafter, leaving the prime responsibility not just for case coordination but also for service provisions with the social services department as the lead agency" (Hallett, 1995, p 215). Even in terms of initial investigation and assessment, the research suggested that the extent of collaboration was largely confined to information exchange and some shared decision making. This was less a case of joint working than of an agreed division of labour with a sequential ordering of tasks being undertaken by separate professions (Birchall with Hallett, 1995). As with the community care experience, it appeared that simply providing the organisational arrangements for interagency collaboration, such as ACPCs and case conferences, was not of itself a guarantee of improved joint working.

Responding to the messages from this research, the DoH embarked in early 1988 on a round of consultation about the content of a new version of the child protection guidance. This asked a series of questions about specific aspects of the child protection process but focused centrally on the general problem of how to ensure wider ownership by agencies other than SSDs. Revealingly, the subtitle of the resulting *Working together to safeguard children* document (DoH et al, 1999) shifted from 'interagency cooperation' to 'interagency working' and reiterated strongly the aims of developing a 'shared responsibility' and an 'integrated approach' on the part of all those involved. As we have seen in Chapter Two, the document also enlarged the range of agencies and professionals potentially at least drawn into the child protection arena, including adult as well as children's services and all aspects of the local authorities' corporate capacity. This guidance was accompanied by a detailed *Framework for the assessment of children in need and their families* (DoH et al, 2000) which aimed to establish a more consistent basis for the judgements of the different professional groups involved.

In addition to detailed practice guidance, the other key way to ensure desired policy outcomes such as effective collaboration is via regulation. In the context of a 'hollowed out' central state, regulation is a way of managing the governance of the 'differentiated polity' that results (see Chapter One). The multiagency nature of child protection work has meant that it has been subject to the involvement of a wide range of regulatory bodies, covering the operation of each of the key constituent agencies. In addition to the Social Services Inspectorate for local authority SSDs and the Audit Commission with responsibility for all public sector services, for example, relevant regulatory bodies include the NHS Executive and its regional offices for the health service; Her Majesty's Inspectorate of Constabulary for the police services; and for education the Office for Standards in Education and Her Majesty's Inspectorate for Education. In addition, the operation of the child protection process is underpinned by the regulatory roles of professional bodies such as the General Medical Council, the Association of Chief Police Officers, the Royal Colleges and the UK Central Council (nursing).

Rather than resolving the problems of 'managing governance', however, there is evidence that the plethora of regulatory mechanisms may hinder the aspirations of 'joined-up' governance. Thus Cope and Goodship (1999) report on a range of 'turf wars' resulting from the different remits, agendas and styles of bodies with overlapping regulatory responsibilities and varying sharpness of 'teeth' (Hughes et al, 1997; also Travers, 1998). In 1996 the Better Regulation Task Force (Burgner, 1996) criticised the largely ad hoc and multifaceted nature of the regulatory system surrounding the operation of the personal social services. The division of responsibilities between different bodies and different professional disciplines was perceived to result in a lack of coherence and consistency, with standards varying between both geographical and service areas. Despite the work of the Social Services Inspectorate, a clear national approach to regulation was seen to be absent. The other main perceived problem was the lack of independence on the part of local and health authorities which were responsible for the regulation and inspection of the services they purchased and/or provided.

The modernisation agenda

The 1998 White Paper *Modernising social services* (DoH, 1998a) set out proposals for strengthening both the guidance given to, and the regulation of, local authority SSDs. The White Paper was part of a wider modernisation agenda on the part of the incoming Labour government which included White Papers on local government (DETR, 1998), the NHS (DoH, 1997), public health (DoH, 1998a) and the *Modernising government* White Paper (Cabinet Office, 1999). As with reform of the public sector undertaken by previous Conservative administrations, the focus of New Labour's modernisation agenda was on effectiveness, efficiency and value for money: "… good quality, best value services, delivering positive outcomes" (DoH, 1998a, p 10). Its declared difference from previous approaches, however, lay in the acceptance by central government of some responsibility for the perceived failures of public sector services and its intention to work in partnership with local authorities: "… to assist local authorities to improve their performance" (1998a, p 10). To this end, the government indicated it would make more explicit than ever before its expectations of the quality of services to be provided by local authorities and of the means by which these expectations would be met: "One big trouble social services has suffered from is that up to now no Government has spelled out exactly what people can expect or what the staff are expected to do. Nor have any clear standards of performance been laid down. This Government is to change all that" (DoH, 1998a, p 2).

Central to the new modernisation agenda was the Labour government's determination to deliver more 'cross-cutting' policy solutions. *Modernising social services* (DoH, 1998a) made very explicit its view that 'user-friendly' services required more extensive collaboration on the part of relevant agencies. Its objective was to foster "… a new spirit of flexible partnership which moves away from sterile conflicts over boundaries" (1998a, p 97). The government was particularly clear about the interdependency of health and social services and about the extent to which greater collaboration was a two-way responsibility. Thus *Modernising social services* stated firmly that the NHS was "… a central partner in almost all social services work" (DoH, 1998a, p 97) and the White Paper on the NHS was equally clear that "…local authorities will be crucial partners in the new approaches to health and health care" (DoH, 1997, p 99). Directors of SSDs would participate in health authority meetings and on the governing bodies of PCGs/PCTs. Further practical expression would be given to this partnership via collaboration in health improvement programmes (HImPs), a key element of which would be the production of joint health and social services investment plans. This greater interdependence was also to apply to the organisational divisions within local authorities. Thus the *Modern local government* White Paper set out a key ambition that authorities "… stop thinking in terms of discrete, departmental function, and start thinking more corporately about what will benefit their citizens, cutting across traditional service boundaries" (DETR, 1998, p 97).

To facilitate this objective, the White Papers proposed a range of 'permissive measures' designed to target some of the traditional barriers to collaboration. *Modernising social services* proposed three key mechanisms to underpin the desired 'partnership in action':

- the ability of local and health authorities to allocate resources into mutually accessible *pooled budgets*, to enable more integrated care;
- arrangements for *lead commissioning*, whereby either health or local authority takes responsibility for purchasing both health and social care, to facilitate the delegation of functions and money;

• the *integrated provision* of health and social care by either agency, to give the NHS greater freedom to deliver social care and enable SSDs to provide some community health services on behalf of the NHS.

These proposals were given legislative form in the 1999 Health Act 'flexibilities', designed to underpin partnerships within local authorities or between them and health authorities, NHS or PCTs. The year 2000 saw the first local authority (the unitary Herefordshire Council) enter a formal partnership arrangement under Section 31 of the Act. Combining the post of social services and housing director with that of the health authority chief executive, the new director is accountable both to local councillors and to the chair of the local health authority.

Modernising social services also set out detailed performance standards for SSDs and the systems for assessing the extent to which they are achieved. A central mechanism was the Best Value initiative. Covering all areas of local government services, Best Value aimed to secure a 'continuous improvement' in services by the introduction of a new, more 'rigorous and systematic' performance framework. This places on local authorities a "... duty to deliver services to clear standards – covering both quality and cost – by the most effective, economic and efficient means possible" (DoH, 1998a, p 113). Under this initiative, local authorities are to carry out fundamental performance reviews of all their services over a five-year cycle, supported by information from a new statistical performance assessment framework (National Best Value Performance Indicators). Specific 'medium-term' targets for health and social care agencies are provided by the National Priorities Guidance and, in children's services, by the *Quality Protects* initiative. The commitment to the interdependence of health and social care services is reflected in the joint nature of the National Priorities Guidance. This guidance identified service sectors that would have a SSD, a NHS or a joint 'lead'. Cutting health inequalities, mental health services and the promotion of independence were designated areas requiring a joint SSD/NHS lead. Although SSDs were to take the lead responsibility for children's welfare, however, the guidance reinforced the message that joint working and the corporate engagement of local authorities was required. Just as SSDs would reflect the HImP objectives in their local plans, so would the NHS and other 'interested parties' be involved in the development of the annual joint children's services plans.

To 'assist' the delivery of reform, the Labour government set out a combination of rewards and sanctions. The performance and assessment framework is underpinned by a 'Modernisation Fund' explicitly to be used as a 'lever for reform'. Payments from the fund are targeted at key areas identified as needing reform and are conditional on effective performance against identified objectives:"... this is not more money to provide more of the same. It is money for change and modernisation. In return for extra public money there must be real improvements in the services given to the public" (DoH, 1998a, p 11). In particular, payment from the Children's Services Grant element of the Social Services Modernisation Fund is dependent on the production and achievement of satisfactory action plans. More punitively, the White Paper makes clear the government's intention to take action against those local authorities not seen to be delivering to required standards: "The government will consider means of rewarding local authorities that are delivering [but] will not hesitate to intervene when services are failing" (1998a, p 118). Those authorities seen to be failing will be required to draw up plans to improve services by a specified date, may be required to accept external management assistance and may, in cases of 'serious service failure', find their responsibilities transferred to another authority or third party.

The 2001 Health and Social Care Bill represented a further extension of the partnership agenda. In contrast to the 1999 Health Act, which accorded considerable autonomy to local agencies, the Health and Social Care Bill introduced the threat of compulsion. Local authorities and health bodies would be directed to pool budgets where voluntary collaboration appeared not to be working. Where services could be seen to have failed, the Bill also proposed the compulsory creation of 'care trusts' to provide all health and social care services to their local populations. The fact that that these trusts would be NHS bodies caused some consternation amongst non-health agencies about the extent to which they would represent a colonisation of social services by the NHS. Last minute concessions, in order to ensure the Bill's passage before the dissolution of Parliament for the 2001 general election, saw the government climb down on the compulsory nature of the care trusts. The determination to enforce better coordination of health and social care services, however, remained undiminished.

The implementation of the government's modernisation agenda is accompanied by a "root and branch reform" of the regulatory system (DoH, 1998a, p 47). A programme of independent inspection is to be developed, underpinned by the new performance framework, incorporating an expanded programme of joint reviews undertaken by the Social Services Inspectorate and the Audit Commission. Eight regional

Commissions for Care Standards (CCSs) are to be established, based on the boundaries of the NHS and social care regions, with a workforce of regional inspectors. Again reinforcing the determination to mandate collaboration, the commissions will comprise representatives of both health and social services and the inspectorate will involve people with skills and qualifications in both fields. The commissions will be independent statutory bodies with their own management boards. Although able to "act in their own right" (DoH, 1998a, p 68), the performance of the CCSs will be monitored by the DoH and will be under the 'direction and guidance' of the Secretary of State.

In children's services, the CCSs will be responsible for inspecting all children's homes, including the voluntary homes previously regulated directly by the DoH, those run by the local authority and those with fewer than four children (previously exempt from registration). All will be subject to mandatory inspection. Independent fostering agencies, state sector boarding schools and residential family centres are also to be brought within this regulatory framework, although there are no plans for the regulation of children's day care services. In addition to regulation via the new CCSs, and to ensure that children's services receive the "closest scrutiny" (DoH, 1998a, p 52), the government has indicated that it will, from 'time to time', commission a single joint report on safeguards for children from all its chief inspectors of services substantially involved with children, including the Office for Standards in Education, the inspectorates for prison, police and probation services, and the Social Services Inspectorate.

Conclusion

Despite more effective collaboration being an enduring social policy aim, this chapter has described how health and social services departments have largely failed to collaborate effectively in either community care or children's services. Commentators argue that this failure derived from a policy focus on the mechanisms and procedures of collaboration rather than on creating the necessary incentives for agencies/professionals to work together. In particular, central policy directives appeared to underestimate the disincentive towards collaboration represented by organisations' fundamental imperative to maintain an orderly and reliable pattern of resource flow (Benson, 1975). In the face of tighter funding controls, and the more competitive context of the health and social care marketplace, key provider organisations arguably became more interested in survival than in cooperation (Salter, 1998).

Collaboration in child protection is especially important given the wide range of agencies and professional groups involved, but it may for the same reason prove particularly difficult to achieve. In response to a series of inquiries highlighting the failure of interagency working, central government has sought to mandate collaboration by means of both regulatory and practice frameworks. As successive drafts of the *Working together* guidance have shifted the ambition from cooperation to collaboration they have become increasingly specific about the mechanisms and procedures designed to underpin joint work at a local level. The collaboration mandate has been considerably strengthened by the 1997 Labour government's wider modernisation agenda that set out to confront some of the traditional barriers to joint working and engender "a new spirit of flexible partnership" (DoH, 1998a, p 97) both between and within health and local authorities.

Earlier chapters have highlighted, however, the potential gap between policy development and its implementation at a local level. Even in a highly prescribed context such as child protection, many factors intervene between policy conception and policy outcome. We have seen how the wider 'sub-structural' imperatives surrounding the behaviour of organisations (in particular the need to secure adequate resources) have undermined the achievement of effective joint working. The central mechanism for reconciling these diverse organisational imperatives in pursuit of a coordinated and coherent local strategy for child protection services is the ACPC. These interagency forums stand at a crucial point between central policy development and local level implementation. The next chapter examines the evidence concerning the nature of the ACPCs and the tensions that surround their key role in child protection.

SEVEN

A system within a system: the role of the Area Child Protection Committee

Introduction

The Area Child Protection Committee (ACPC) is a joint forum comprising representatives of a wide range of agencies and professional groups working together in child protection. Its central role is to underpin interagency collaboration by developing, monitoring and reviewing local policies and procedures. Functioning as a middle layer between the broad frameworks of central government policy and the specific protocols of local level practice, the ACPC has been described as a 'system within a system': "... the co-ordinating body of the local child protection system ... operating within the external 'system' of government child protection policy" (Sanders, 1999, p 264). As such it can be seen as a central mechanism for delivering the mandated coordination of local child protection networks.

As we have argued, the achievement of ideological/domain consensus, effective work coordination and mutual positive evaluation between participants are important prerequisites of effective interagency cooperation. We have seen in earlier chapters how these 'superstructural' attributes can be affected by different organisational imperatives surrounding network participants (sub-structural factors). Threats to collaboration on the above dimensions may arise from tensions deriving from any or all of four central aspects of those agencies' wider objectives: fulfilment of central service delivery requirements; maximisation of public support/legitimacy for the service agenda; achievement of orderly and reliable patterns of key resources; and defence of operational paradigms (the 'technological–ideological commitment' to certain ways of working). As Benson argues: "Consensus between agencies on matters of domain and ideology can ... only occur within limits set by their market positions"

(1975, p 237). Within a multiagency forum like the ACPC, the wider interests of participating organisations may constrain not only the representatives' ability to make certain decisions (especially if they carry financial implications) within the ACPC, but may also affect the implementation of any ACPC decisions at operational level.

The following section will describe the composition of the ACPC, exploring in particular the extent and nature of participation by health managers and professionals. After examining changing government expectations surrounding ACPC operation, the chapter will assess the extent to which it is able effectively to operate as a mechanism for mandated coordination within the local child protection process. In doing so, the chapter will draw on the relatively small number of empirical studies (from primary or secondary data) of the ACPC's operation (Jackson et al, 1994; Hallett, 1995; Armstrong, 1995, 1996; Sanders et al, 1997) including a large-scale investigation undertaken by the authors between 1996 and 1998 (Lupton et al, 1999b). This last study involved in-depth interviews with strategic and front-line staff in three case study sites as well as a postal survey of the views of ACPC members across the South West of England (see Introduction for details). It should be noted that all these studies were undertaken in the period between the 1991 and 1999 versions of the *Working together* guidance.

The ACPC composition

As described in Chapter Two, successive versions of the *Working together* guidance attempted to draw more players into the ACPC arena. In addition to an extended list of key agencies, the government's determination to achieve more 'cross-cutting' services for children and families saw the 1999 guidance providing an extensive catalogue of other agencies with which the ACPC is to develop 'appropriate arrangements'. These include: adult, child and adolescent mental health services; sexual health and drug and alcohol misuse services; the Crown Prosecution Service; coroner, judiciary and local authority legal services; prison, youth detention/ offending services; and representatives of service users and their carers. Although the question of greater central prescription of the ACPC membership was raised in advance of its publication, the 1999 guidance retained the position that actual membership should be left to local determination. Reflecting in part the concern to legitimise existing practice in some localities, however, but also the desire to ensure greater 'ownership' of ACPC decisions on the part of participating agencies, the

1999 guidance established that the chair of the ACPC could be drawn from any member agency, may rotate between agencies, or may be assumed by someone "… of sufficient standing and expertise" from outside the ACPC (DoH et al, 1999, p 36).

Research undertaken in the early 1990s in Wales (Jackson et al, 1994) indicated that the actual membership of ACPCs appeared fairly closely to reflect central guidance. The following agencies were represented on all ACPCs surveyed: social services (senior manager and child protection coordinator); health (nursing, child psychiatry and paediatrics); education (Local Education Authority); police (senior police officer); probation; and the NSPCC. Representatives from other agencies or professional groups such as the police surgeons, the Crown Prosecution Service, the school medical service and racial equality councils were each found in only one of the eight ACPCs studied. The size of the ACPCs ranged considerably, with the largest involving just over three times as many members as the smallest. The larger committees included some of the other agencies (such as adult psychiatric services and voluntary agencies) with which the guidance had recommended establishing links, and the smaller ones had no representation from some of those agencies listed as central (for example, GPs, teachers). Sanders et al (1997) revealed a close relationship between the size of the ACPC and agency attendance, with smaller ACPCs generally ensuring more frequent attendance on the part of their members.

In respect of the NHS more specifically, the same study found a preponderance of health representatives on ACPCs, even over social services, with three NHS members for every two from SSDs. The numerical dominance of health members is confirmed by Lupton et al (1999b), although this study also reveals considerable diversity in terms of both the site and nature of NHS representation. With the exception of the low level of GP attendance (confirmed by Armstrong, 1995), neither study reported any widespread concern about the level or nature of NHS representation. However, Lupton et al (1999b) identified a majority view on the part of NHS and non-NHS representatives alike that a balance had to be struck between obtaining sufficient representation from all key aspects of the NHS and ensuring that the ACPC was not thereby dominated by NHS staff:

> "I think health needs to sort out their representation on the ACPC because health is a complex, massive organisation. There are so many different bits to health, and I think other agencies don't realise that.

They think that health is one big blob and that they all talk to each other, but they don't.... I think health has to sort out what they are going to do with their designated doctors and nurses and [their] management input and how the two are going to sit together. So health needs to sort out their ACPC representation and that needs to be negotiated in the context of what is the right size of the committee in terms of being effective, not being so big that it's unmanageable. Within that health needs to decide,'... Well, can this person speak for all of us?' You would have to have meetings the size of Wembley Stadium to have a complete representation of health – it would be health rent-a-mob." (social services manager, case study site, Lupton et al, 1999b, p 27)

The role of the ACPC

As described in Chapter Two, the ACPCs were initially established in 1974 as Area Review Committees (ARCs) with a brief to develop and advise on local systems for interagency work and to provide interagency training. Following the Cleveland inquiry, the 1988 *Working together* guidance required the renamed ACPCs to review the 'significant issues' arising from local agencies' investigations of child abuse cases and to oversee both preventative work and interagency liaison (DoH, 1998b). The 1991 revision of the guidance set out a more proactive role on the part of the committees (Hallett, 1995), replacing the responsibility to 'review' with the requirement to 'scrutinise' local practice and, where necessary,"... make recommendations to the responsible agencies" (Home Office et al, 1991, p 5). This document also saw a further extension of the ACPC role in terms of monitoring the implementation of local procedures, conducting a 'composite' review of any case involving a child fatality ('Part 8' case review) and publishing an annual report of its activities.

Although promoting a more proactive approach on the part of the ACPC, the 1991 guidance stopped short of giving the ACPCs a remit to develop specific protocols for local interagency practice (Sanders, 1999). Evidence was increasing, however, of variability in the extent to which ACPCs sought or achieved consistency in local practice (SSI, 1995; SSI Wales, 1996). The analysis by Sanders et al (1997) revealed a close relationship between the extent of prescription in the guidance and the degree of latitude exercised by the ACPC in respect of variations in local practice: "... the less specific and comprehensive the interagency child protection guidance, the more ACPCs would appear to either tolerate wide variations in practice or else be prepared to find other means of ensuring consistency of practice" (1999, p 123). By the 1999 version of the guidance, therefore, we find that the relatively laissez-faire approach had given way to a determination to achieve more uniformity and consistency in local practice. There was evident a stronger determination to use the ACPCs more explicitly as a mechanism for mandated coordination. Whereas previously the ACPCs had been given fairly broad parameters in respect of, for example, the conduct of 'Part 8' case reviews or the provision of local interagency training, the 1999 guidance contained specific proposals for the discharge of these responsibilities.

The main change between the 1991 and 1999 versions of the central guidance, however, was the incorporation of the ACPCs into new national performance and planning frameworks. In particular, as set out in Chapter Six, the ACPCs would now be required to work within the framework established by the local interagency children's services plan to deliver more coordinated provision for children in need and those requiring protection. Each would produce an annual business plan, including 'measurable objectives' (DoH et al, 1999, p 37) that would both derive from and in turn contribute to the children's services plans. In addition ACPCs were given an extended mandate to ensure a 'level of agreement and understanding' across local agencies about operational definitions and thresholds for intervention. Achievement of this understanding was to be underpinned by a new national *Framework for the assessment of children in need and their families* (DoH et al, 2000).

Coalition or federation?

Hallett (1995) cites a number of typologies of interagency working from the loosest forms of communication or informal 'mutual adjustment', through a range of more routinised forms of cooperation or 'alliance', to the most formal 'corporate' strategies and ultimately to full 'merger'. Further distinction is made within the broad 'alliance' strategy between the 'coalition' (informal authority system, with power being retained by individual organisations and no sanctions for non-participation) and the 'federation'. The latter typically involves a supra-organisational administrative authority: "When the organisations are willing to define the goals and tasks and when they are willing to cede a degree of their autonomy to that joint structure" (Davidson, 1976, quoted in Hallett, 1995, p 275). The assumption underpinning these continua is that joint working is likely to be easier and more effective the closer the structure is to the federation model.

Hallett (1995) considers that ACPCs are located somewhere between the coalition and federation stages, given that there is a formal structure and the central guidance represents an (increasing) attempt to regulate their operational autonomy. While there may be considerable informal pressure to cooperate in the ACPC, however, there is no formal sanction for non-participation. Nevertheless, with the establishment of their own budgets and the ability to appoint staff, Hallett argues, the ACPCs moved closer to the 'federation' end of the continuum. As Armstrong (1995) comments: "With staff to initiate and progress the work, ACPCs achieve a power of direct action that otherwise often eludes them" (1995, p 21). Subsequent evidence, however, suggests that the extent of this power may be extremely limited; effectively constrained by the inability of ACPCs to override the more pressing central objectives of participating organisations. Central among these objectives is the organisational requirement to secure and defend core resources.

Defence of core resources

The 1991 guidance enabled ACPCs to make arrangements with their constituent agencies to establish an annual budget to support the work of the committee's secretariat and any joint training activity. Subsequent evidence indicates that the nature and level of both financial support and staffing for the ACPCs has been extremely variable (Armstrong, 1995). Hallett (1995) highlighted a concern on the part of ACPC members about lack of funding and the view that more specific apportionment of costs was necessary between agencies, especially for those who participated in more than one ACPC. The later study by Lupton et al (1999b) revealed a general perception that inadequate funding restricted the ability of ACPCs to effect the required policy and practice developments within their constituent agencies.

While the consultation on the 1999 guidance invited views on ways to strengthen financial support to ACPCs, there was no suggestion that government funds would be provided to support their operation nor that funding should be guaranteed to a minimum level. The finance and administration of the ACPCs was to remain a 'matter for local agreement', subject only to the admonition that: "As a multi-agency forum, the ACPC should be supported in its work by its main constituent agencies" (DoH et al, 1999, p 36).

Lupton et al's study indicates that the issue of resources may place considerable strain on collaborative working. In the face of budgetary constraints, organisations were seen to be reluctant to accept financial responsibility for additional service developments, particularly in preventative work:

> "Lack of resources has a role to play because, as resources get tight, people tend to draw back into their organisational/professional shells to protect what they've got rather than saying that, if we put everything together, could we provide better services ... but people aren't generally willing to say that...." (NHS trust manager, case study site, Lupton et al, 1999b)

In turn, such financial considerations were seen to constrain the ability of organisational representatives to take the relevant decisions within the ACPC. Thus Jackson et al (1994) conclude that, while ACPC representatives generally perceived they could agree on decisions about matters of practice, training or local guidance, they were less likely to feel that they could commit their agencies to financial decisions or policy changes. In addition, even if willing to take such decisions, Lupton et al (1999b) report the view that agencies' ability to do so is inhibited by different financial and planning cycles:

> "I think that if you are operating at the optimum in terms of joint planning and commissioning, those bits of the planning cycle need to be in tandem with one another in order for that to occur, but there needs to be ... some power shift in terms of people being able to make those decisions at a particular time." (child protection ACPC advisor, case study site, Lupton et al, 1999b)

Work coordination

In order to strengthen the authority of the ACPC, the *Working together* guidance stresses the importance of its members' status. If it is to influence the actions of participating agencies, it is important that the ACPC comprises members of sufficient authority: "... to allow them to speak on their agencies' behalf and to make decisions to an agreed level without referral to the appointees' agencies. The level of decision-making delegated to appointees needs to be considerable to enable ACPCs to operate effectively" (Home Office et al, 1991, p 6, para 2.8). Particularly from health and education services, however, there is evidence that ACPCs have found it difficult to attract representatives of sufficient seniority to make budgetary decisions, to ensure effective feedback on or implementation of ACPC policies or to demonstrate ownership of ACPC business (Hallett, 1995). Around half of the ACPC respondents in Lupton et al's study felt that, as a result, their ACPC operated as an information-giving, rather than a decision-making, forum. Interestingly, this was more likely to be the view of NHS than non-NHS respondents. As Sanders et al (1997) point out, there is no necessary correspondence between managerial level and the ability to make delegated decisions. Some members of non-senior rank nevertheless had sufficient delegated authority to make key decisions. A particular problem, however, is presented by those members, such as GPs and local head teachers, who lack the 'corporate capacity' to represent anyone other than themselves.

Lupton et al's study also suggests, however, that there may be a tension within ACPCs between having members with sufficient seniority to make decisions on the one hand and having staff with the ability to effect change at the operational level on the other. Under half of all regional respondents, for example, indicated that they routinely fed back on ACPC matters to operational levels within their organisations and the majority considered that they were only able to achieve local change 'to an extent'. Again, difficulties in this respect may be particularly true of NHS members. Thus, NHS survey respondents were markedly less likely than their non-NHS colleagues to feel that the ACPC was able to effect operational change and the view of many non-NHS representatives was that health members were the main problem in this respect:

> "Health purchasers seem to be the main stumbling block for us – other agencies seem to be able to effect operational change." (non-NHS ACPC member, regional survey, Lupton et al, 1999b)

A large minority view, particularly articulated by the designated NHS personnel, was that greater participation by front-line professionals would improve the likelihood of effective decision making within the ACPC and of those decisions being implemented at the operational level.

Lupton et al (1999b) found respondents fairly evenly divided on the question of whether the effectiveness of the ACPC would be improved by giving it statutory powers, with little difference being evident between NHS and non-NHS respondents on this issue. For those in favour, a statutory basis was seen to increase the likelihood that the ACPC could reach over into participating organisations and ensure the implementation of its decisions:

> "Statutory status would mean that actions/agreements must be enforced which would probably improve effectiveness and outcomes and nobody could slide out of their commitments." (NHS ACPC member, regional survey, Lupton et al, 1999b)

Those against the idea considered that it would be impossible to achieve, given the fact that its members must ultimately remain accountable to their own agencies. Yet others felt that, even if it were possible, it would be undesirable to increase the power and authority of the ACPC over its participating agencies. Perhaps not surprisingly, this latter view was particularly likely to be offered by NHS respondents:

> "Statutory status is two-edged. The ACPC could become a quango and would certainly suffer if [it was] without a commensurate budget. But a budget would increase the risk of quango status." (NHS ACPC member, regional survey, Lupton et al, 1999b)

In the consultation process on the 1999 guidance, the issue of placing ACPCs on a statutory footing was raised, only to be effectively foreclosed with the comment that: "... the government doubts that the arguments for placing the work of ACPCs on a statutory footing are compelling" (DoH, 1998b, p 10). Perhaps not surprisingly the outcome of the consultation process recommended the continuation of the status quo. Area Child Protection Committee members are accountable to their parent organisations, which must agree any actions with policy or resource implications. The subsequent guidance, however, considered that the development of more extensive national performance frameworks would help ensure agreement within participating agencies: "Programmes of work should be agreed and endorsed at a senior level within each of the member agencies, within the framework of the children's services plan" (DoH et al, 1999, p 34).

Domain consensus

Arguably, a central prerequisite of the ACPC's effective operation is that participating agencies share a sense of 'ownership' of the committee and its decisions. As with the 'inner' and 'outer' layers of the front-line provider networks, however, evidence suggests that ACPCs experience by varying degrees of involvement on the part of their agency members. Thus Sanders et al (1997) argued that 'full ownership' of the ACPC may only really be characteristic of SSD staff and, to an extent, the police. Representatives of these two agencies are most likely to attend the ACPC and to contribute to its agenda. This appears to be reinforced by Hallett's (1995) finding that only members from social services and the police perceived they exerted a 'great deal' of influence over the ACPC. Community nurses, probation officers, teachers and clinical medical officers generally recorded 'a modest amount' of influence and those claiming to have only 'a little' influence included child psychiatrists and school representatives (1995, p 282). Despite the interagency composition of ACPCs, Lupton et al (1999b) found that the great majority of both health and non-health respondents considered that the committees were in effect 'led by social services':

> "... the length of meetings and the dominance of social services related issues prevents the involvement of other professionals who would have a great deal to contribute towards child protection issues." (NHS ACPC member, regional survey, Lupton et al, 1999b)

Sanders et al (1997) argue that the sense of involvement in, or ownership of, the ACPC is related to the extent of match between the ACPC's core agenda and the policies and priorities of participating agencies. Official emphasis given to the procedures surrounding investigation, they suggest, means that agencies such as social services and the police, and to an extent some health professionals such as paediatricians, are likely to play a significant role in the ACPC itself, as well as in the operation of its sub-groups. In comparison, agencies or groups such as other health professionals, education, probation and so on, who are traditionally more concerned with prevention and treatment, may feel increasingly marginalised in discussions focusing on the procedures surrounding investigation (recognition, referral, conferencing and registration/deregistration). The finding of Jackson et al (1994) that many ACPC members found the focus on the 'forensic process' of investigating abuse too constraining is echoed by the more recent study by Lupton et al (1999b) where the majority of both NHS and non-NHS respondents considered that the ACPC was over-concerned with investigative procedures at the expense of broader child welfare approaches. The more peripheral the level of their involvement, the more likely it will be that these groups will experience dissonance surrounding, and (perceived at least) devaluation of, their role within the ACPC.

Ideological consensus and positive evaluation

Arguably one central function of central guidance is to mitigate differences in work coordination by strengthening the degree of domain (who does what) and ideological consensus (how do they do it) within local networks. In turn this should encourage greater mutual positive evaluation (how well they do it) on the part of their diverse participants. Via the production of local level protocols and procedures, the role of the ACPC is potentially crucial in this respect. Hallett's (1995) study revealed that the ACPC was seen to function best in "… establishing, maintaining and reviewing interagency procedures" (p 336) and Sanders et al (1997) conclude that the procedural handbooks were very effective in ensuring that investigation took place "… within a policy context, thereby ensuring consistency of practice" (p 124).

Lupton et al's study, however, indicates that there may be differences between NHS and non–NHS professionals in terms of their susceptibility to pressures towards greater interdisciplinary consensus. The regional survey of ACPC members, for example, indicates that non–NHS members, especially from SSDs, were generally positive about the attempt to develop common procedures and agreed ways of working. In contrast, health members were more likely to feel that the child protection process had become 'overly proceduralised' and constraining of professional judgement:

> "They are a useful framework for health professionals, but are not a substitute for clinical knowledge and expertise." (NHS ACPC member, regional survey, Lupton et al, 1999b)

Related to the view that social services' agendas and concerns tended to dominate the ACPC was the perception that the procedures emanating from the ACPC were in effect those of the SSD:

> "Social services have their procedures (decided on unilaterally) which bind everyone else, yet at the same time ensure that no one gets heard." (NHS ACPC member, regional survey, Lupton et al, 1999b)

If the impact of the ACPC appears mixed in respect of encouraging greater ideological consensus, evidence suggests that it may make an important contribution in respect of engendering positive evaluation. Lupton et al (1999b) found that the ACPCs were generally seen to be successful in encouraging a greater mutual appreciation of the roles of, and constraints experienced by, colleagues from other agencies. Their study revealed both NHS and non-NHS members rating highly the ability of the ACPC to improve the understanding of each agency's role in child protection, and qualitative comments indicated a widespread view that the ACPCs enabled a better appreciation of the situation of other agencies:

> "I think that clarity of each other's roles has got better as the ACPC has developed. I think the appreciation of each other's agendas has got better and some of the difficulties the ACPC has gone through has eliminated those different problems and different agendas." (ACPC chair, case study site, Lupton et al, 1999b)

Impact of exogenous change

As Hallett (1995) has argued, the mechanisms for interagency collaboration in child protection were developed in the context of relatively uniform and predictable public state welfare services. Since the mid-1980s, however, the public sector has been subject to a radical and ongoing process of restructuring, with major implications for the operation of existing multiagency networks. There is evidence that two areas of change in particular may have impacted on the work of the ACPCs: the ongoing restructuring of the NHS, with the creation of the purchaser/provider division and the shift towards primary-based care and, more locally, the further round of local government reorganisation which took place in 1996/97.

At its most basic, the existence of a multiplicity of purchasers and providers (some of whom are independent) makes the job of coordinating the planning and provision of services more difficult. Lupton et al (1999b) found a general perception that the creation of internal markets within the public sector had hindered effective interagency collaboration and that the fragmentation of the NHS had particularly affected the role of health professionals. The problem of physical fragmentation was seen to have been exacerbated by the (then) competitive ethos of the internal market. Respondents commented on the way in which they felt a more market-driven approach had worked against the development of shared goals and priorities by increasing budgetary protectionism and introducing conflicting agendas between purchasers and providers:

> "I think the marketplace has damaged child protection work, it has made everyone think very competitively, and think of the business opportunities within their own organisation, rather than looking at child protection issues.... I think purchasers and providers have different agendas generally. Purchasers are anxious to look at the services which need to be provided; providers are concerned about how it is going to be resourced. They are very difficult to reconcile sometimes." (named nurse, case study site, Lupton et al, 1999b)

Lupton et al's study was undertaken at the inception of the new PCGs/PCTs and respondents were mixed in their anticipation about the way in which these new structures would affect the operation of the ACPCs. Overall, NHS respondents were less sure than their non-NHS colleagues about their impact but those who had a view tended to be more pessimistic. Whereas exactly one third of non-NHS members agreed with the statement that the formation of PCG/PCTs would improve interagency working in child protection, this was the view of only one quarter of NHS members. The general view was that much would depend on the way in which the PCGs approached their role:

> "PCGs should be a great opportunity for improving local care. However, a countywide perspective may be lost as a consequence. How PCGs liaise with DHAs, local authorities and a countywide ACPC remains to be seen." (consultant paediatrician, regional survey, Lupton et al, 1999b)

The impact of local government reorganisation in contrast had already been felt by many of the ACPCs in Lupton et al's study and the reaction was generally mixed. On the one hand, it was clear that local government reorganisation had exacerbated problems of coterminosity, with respondents expressing concerns about workload implications for agencies which, as a result, now had to attend more than one ACPC. Concerns were also voiced, particularly on the part of NHS members, about the difficulty of working with several ACPCs that had developed different local guidelines and systems. There was also a perception that the process of change exacerbated the tendency of organisations to prioritise their own concerns and increased the likelihood of communication difficulties:

"... any organisational change affects the dynamics of an organisation, therefore you have to manage those dynamics within the context of change to ensure that child protection keeps on happening. The tendency will be to focus on the needs of the organisations. If you look at any of the inquiries in which reorganisation has been a factor, they do demonstrate that they tend to breakdown communication because people are busy changing." (ACPC child protection advisor, case study, Lupton et al, 1999b)

In contrast, non-health ACPC members, particularly those in the new unitary authorities, were generally positive about the changes. For these respondents, the initial disruption caused by local government reorganisation was seen to be more than outweighed by the potential benefits of developing more locally focused child protection policies:

"Now we have the opportunity of meeting our very specific needs." (senior SSD manager, new unitary case study site, Lupton et al, 1999b)

Overall, however, there was evident a fairly widespread view that the assumptions of central policy guidance did not sufficiently take into account the work coordination implications of organisational change:

"You have documents from the DoH which don't account for all these organisational changes, which assumes that things are just the way they were before these changes. So it is hardly surprising that there's a gap between what the strategists are hoping to do and what those who are doing the job actually do." (NSPCC manager, case study site, Lupton et al, 1999b)

Conclusion

We have argued that, as an interagency coordinating committee, the ACPC is an important mechanism in the mandated cooperation of local child protection networks. Described as "a system within a system" (Sanders, 1999, p 264), the ACPC represents a key layer between the development of policy and its implementation at a local level. Over the years the operation of the ACPC has been subject to increased central prescription as various versions of government guidance have sought to enhance its role within local provider networks. In particular, improvement in the ability of the ACPC to engender greater coherence and consistency in local interagency practice has been sought via its incorporation within national performance management and assessment frameworks and by efforts to increase the multiagency ownership of its operation. The provision of its own budget and the ability to appoint staff, some argue, has given the ACPC greater power of direct action over the practices of its constituent agencies.

However, the chapter has also outlined evidence of significant constraints, both internal and external, over the ACPC's development of a more proactive role within local networks. One particular constraint is the limited extent to which the ACPC is able to determine the relevant actions of its constituent agencies. Despite their seniority, many ACPC members feel unable to make decisions on behalf of their agencies, particularly if those decisions carry financial or other resource implications. The effective implementation of its policies, moreover, seems limited by the uneven nature of the relationship between the ACPC and front-line staff. In addition, the evidence suggests that the effectiveness of the ACPC may be inhibited by a range of practical difficulties in work coordination (especially financial and planning cycles) between its member agencies. Rather than the ACPC being the cement that holds these agencies together in times of external change, it appears that central guidance may underestimate the extent to which these changes, particularly in respect of creation of public sector markets and local government reorganisation, have adversely affected the basis of collaboration within the ACPC. Although successful in encouraging mutual positive evaluation on the part of its members, ACPCs appear to have experienced less success in increasing the degree of ideological consensus on the part of its diverse member agencies and professional groups.

The available evidence suggests that the experience and contribution of the NHS within the ACPC may be particularly problematic. The increased fragmentation of the health service has affected both the nature of its representation on the ACPC and the ability of its staff to participate effectively therein. Although present in significant numbers, the extent to which NHS members feel centrally involved in the operation of the ACPC seems to be variable. Despite government efforts to increase its multiagency ownership, many NHS members appear still to experience the ACPC as dominated by the agendas and concerns of SSDs. The only limited commitment of NHS staff to the development of common procedures and protocols for professional practice must be seen in this light, as well as due to the resistance of many medical professionals to the process of codification and routinisation that such procedures represent (see Chapter Three). Partly as a result of these particular difficulties, NHS members are seen to be among the ACPC members least able to effect change at local level. Recognition of some of the dilemmas for the NHS role in child protection as a result of its organisational fragmentation was one motivation behind the creation of the designated and named health professional posts. The next chapter examines in greater depth the experience and impact of these key NHS professionals within local child provider networks.

EIGHT

Agents of change? The role of the designated and named health professionals

Introduction

Earlier chapters have begun to indicate the extent of change required to bring about improvements in collaboration within interprofessional networks. Attempts to facilitate change in the commercial sector highlight the importance of introducing a specialist position of 'champion' or 'agent' of change. This individual is responsible for encouraging staff to engage in best practice and to work collaboratively across disciplinary, organisational and cultural boundaries in the pursuit of mutual interests (Crane, 1998; Davenport and Prusack, 1998). In the child protection context, the introduction of the designated and named doctor/nurse roles can be seen as a means of developing this change agent role.

There are two interrelated roles undertaken by change agents. One may be described as that of the 'knowledge champion', and this role has received considerable attention in the growing body of knowledge management literature. The acquisition of new knowledge and its transfer among workers is increasingly seen as a critical corporate attribute, central to the pursuit of competitive advantage (Blackler, 1995). Organisations are exhorted by management theorists to tackle dysfunctional actions like knowledge hoarding, inertia or resistance to new knowledge by creating a specific position of 'chief knowledge officer' (Davenport and Prusak, 1998; Duke et al, 1999) or 'knowledge manager"(Ichijo et al, 1998) to lead their corporate knowledge strategy.

Drawing on this literature, the tasks of knowledge champions can be delineated as being to:

• collate and distribute already explicit knowledge in accessible formats;

- exhort or cajole staff to engage in knowledge sharing and drop their resistance to new knowledge or ways of working;
- serve as a 'human interface' by passing issues from the field up to management levels;
- develop training content and the technologies to make it accessible and utilised;
- serve as the central focal point for knowledge use and sharing by providing 'help-desk' support and structured debriefings;
- coordinate and manage learning and knowledge-sharing initiatives; and
- encourage discursive reflection on actions and reactions.

Whereas these efforts are largely 'internal' in terms of building the necessary technological and cultural infrastructure to foster innovation between different disciplines/tiers *within* organisations, they may also involve relationships with other organisations. Change agents in this latter sense can thus also be 'cultural mediators', helping to develop common meaning and understanding *across* organisational and cultural boundaries. This role involves identifying and managing areas of conflict, sharing perspectives, and information exchange (Crane, 1998; Caddick et al, 1999; Schmitz, 2000). Crane's (1998) study of business–non-governmental organisations (NGOs) collaborative initiatives found that success often depended on certain key individuals and groups within the alliance:

> … translators of cultural knowledge between cultural and subcultural groups, providing shared vocabularies and frames of reference, such that cultural clash did not impose impossible obstacles for effective communication to take place and for mutual respect and understanding to be fostered. (Crane, 1998, p 72)

The knowledge-giving and bridging role of change agents can positively impact on the operation of interprofessional networks in child protection, in so far as they contribute towards the development of ideological and domain consensus, mutual evaluation and improved work coordination across disciplinary and organisational boundaries.

This chapter begins by assessing the 'change agent' potential of the named and designated health professional roles. Drawing on recent empirical evidence, it identifies a number of constraints surrounding the effective performance of these roles in child protection. These constraints, it argues, serve further to illuminate some of the wider tensions characterising the operation of interprofessional and multiagency networks, in particular those arising around issues of representation and accountability.

The designated and named roles

The identification of recurrent failures in professional practice in the two major overviews of child protection inquiry reports (DHSS, 1982; DoH, 1991) alerted policy makers to the inadequacies of arrangements for the management, support and training of staff in agencies such as health and education. The two studies highlighted the need for staff, in particular health professionals, to have access to senior co-workers within their workplace who are sufficiently knowledgeable of, and experienced in, the subject of child abuse. These staff could offer supervision, training and expert advice to colleagues, as well as liaise effectively with staff in other agencies. Recommendations arising from these inquiries were instrumental in the designation of a specialist doctor and nurse role in the 1988 version of the *Working together* guidance DHSS and Welsh Office, 1988, paras 5.50-5.33). Further description of these roles was offered in two addenda: *Diagnosis of child sexual abuse: Guidance for doctors* (DHSS, 1988a) and *Guidance for senior nurses, health visitors, and midwives* (DHSS, 1988b), produced by members of the Medical and Nursing Standing Advisory Committees to the Secretary of State.

Subsequent guidance was issued to take into account recommendations from new inquiries, new knowledge about child abuse and the more inclusive framework for the care and protection of children established by the 1989 Children Act (*Child protection: Medical responsibilities: Guidance to doctors working with child protection agencies*, DoH, 1996, and *Child protection: Guidance for senior nurses, health visitors and midwives*, DoH, 1992b). Wider policy changes were also to have a major influence on the development of the named and designated roles. The cascade of health service reforms initiated by the 1989 NHS and Community Care Act radically altered working arrangements within the NHS in the early part of the 1990s, in particular diversifying service responsibilities and creating new and independent management tiers. At one level, the decentralisation of the health service exacerbated the practical difficulties of implementing the quasi-regulatory framework of child protection procedures and protocols and placed a premium on greater coordination across service providers. At another level, it necessitated clarification of the respective responsibilities of those commissioning and those providing health services.

In the context of wider policy changes, coupled with the absence of a statutory framework to ensure policy compliance, the appointment of designated doctors and nurses represented a means of improving the coordination of child protection activities across the NHS and of tracking and monitoring implementation. These functions are evident in the expanding remit of the roles in successive versions of the *Working together* guidance. The recommendation in the 1988 guidance that health authorities "… identify a doctor and senior nurse to coordinate the provision of advice to SSDs" (DHSS and Welsh Office, 1988, p 6) was extended in the 1991 guidance to the appointment of a senior doctor, a senior nurse with a health visiting qualification and a senior midwife.

The proposed duties of these 'designated' posts were also expanded. Their role was now to ensure child protection policies were in place for health staff; to set up effective communication systems to coordinate work; to take responsibility for identifying training needs and providing clinical instruction; to coordinate all aspects of child protection work within their health district; to provide advice to health professionals and social services on all aspects of child protection; and to work with other agencies on the development of interagency procedures. The last role assigned designated health professionals to local interagency forums such as Area Child Protection Committees (ACPCs). A new addendum to the guidance in 1995 identified the additional role of the 'named' health professional (DoH and Welsh Office, 1995). Employed by the provider trusts, the named staff were to be more proactive at the operational level, assisting designating professionals in the day-to-day monitoring and provision of advice, support and training to staff on child protection matters. The most recent revision of the guidance (DoH et al, 1999) enhances the remit of the named role, giving incumbents the lead responsibility for child protection within health provider units.

The publication of the 1991 *Working together* guidance (Home Office et al, 1991) came just before the health service reforms began to take effect and thus did not address the implications of the internal market. Designated professionals would normally be *employed by* the health provider trust but would be *appointed by* the commissioning health authority. It was not until 1995 that further guidance (*Child protection: Clarification of agreements between the NHS and other agencies*, DoH and Welsh Office, 1995) was provided in respect of the health service and its constituent professional/service divisions. This continued to rest accountability for the delivery of the health component of child protection on the health authority, but was hazy on the question of how designated professionals would be represented on, and held accountable within, the ACPC.

In view of the responsibilities described above, it can be argued that designated and named professionals, potentially at least, perform an important function as change agents within the NHS. They are important providers, enablers and integrators of knowledge pertaining to child abuse and child protection. They are also responsible for training provision across a diversity of health settings, from general practice to dentistry, and are thus well positioned to initiate shared learning methods. Contact with a wide range of different professional groups at the field level, moreover, arguably affords the designated and named personnel the opportunity to work on the interpersonal dimensions of collaboration, providing support to colleagues undertaking stressful child protection work. Their role could thus enable practitioners to express frustrations and emotions as well as to identify professional capabilities, motivations and interests in respect of child protection work. These could then be relayed to strategic level staff in order to ensure that local policy making reflects 'real life' working contexts. In particular, the involvement of designated health professionals in interagency forums like the ACPC places them in a position to clarify the respective roles and responsibilities of different health professional groups for those outside the NHS and to present the 'health perspective' on local child protection issues.

Designated and named professionals in practice

Assessment of the roles of designated and named staff is hampered by the paucity of empirical evidence surrounding their performance. As such, what follows draws heavily on a study undertaken by the authors (Lupton et al, 1999b) in the South West of England towards the end of the 1990s. As well as interviews with strategic personnel (both NHS and non-NHS, n=67) across three local authority sites and a survey of ACPC members across the South West region (n=140) this included in-depth interviews with designated (n=7) and named (n=12) health professionals themselves (see Introduction for further details). The study revealed considerable variations in the contractual arrangements for the appointment of designated and named staff across the three health authorities and identified a number of tensions surrounding the performance of the roles, including issues of role clarity, representation and accountability, work coordination and resources.

Appointment of posts

A consistent feature in all health authorities was the variable time taken to appoint the designated and named positions. In the initial phase of the investigation, which took place in 1996, Lupton and her colleagues found only one authority where a designated and named nurse had been in post for more than two years. In another health authority, a doctor described himself as being in the named position "... on and off for about six years". With these exceptions, the named and designated personnel were fairly newly appointed. All health authorities reported particular difficulties in recruiting designated doctors, with the result that posts were left vacant for some time. One reason for this difficulty appeared to be the perception on the part of senior doctors that the role would entail additional work and provide inadequate remuneration. Differences between the salaries of senior doctors and senior nurses meant that considerably less difficulty was experienced in recruiting the designated nurse personnel.

Professional expertise and training

A central prerequisite of the change agent role is that incumbents should be highly knowledgeable, experienced and adequately trained in order that they can provide informed advice to colleagues. The designated and named health professionals interviewed by Lupton and colleagues were all found to have received some form of professional education or training in identifying the signs and symptoms of abuse and in the aetiology of child abuse. Only 4 out of the 7 designated professionals, however, and only 3 out of the 12 named professionals had received the interagency child protection training jointly administered by the local authority SSD and the police authority. Two designated doctors reported that they had been given no further post-qualification training in the management of child protection and this was true for all three named doctors and two of the named nurses. The remaining nurse professional had received training via a range of sources, from courses provided by the NSPCC to those delivered by the local school of nursing.

The lack of interagency training left some of the named health professionals feeling 'out on a limb', a perception compounded, in their view, by their relative lack of experience in child protection work. While half of the named health professionals described their previous experience in child protection as 'very substantial', the remainder categorised their

Table 1: Self-evaluation by designated and named health professionals of their child protection experience

Extent	Designated [n=7]	Named [n=12]
Very substantial	5	6
Quite substantial	0	3
Not very substantial	2	3

experience as either 'quite substantial' or 'not very substantial' (see Table 1). The self-perceived experience of the designated staff appeared generally greater. As a counterbalance to the lack of specialist training/interagency training, most named health professionals felt that informal supervisory sessions with designated health professionals and ward managers had provided a useful way of acquiring new knowledge. In addition, such contact was valued as a support mechanism to help allay some of the anxiety entailed in child protection work.

Accountability

A few designated health professionals reported confusion about professional accountability, given the separation between the provider trusts which employ them and the health authority which funds their designated role. A designated nurse articulated this tension in the following way:

> "I think there is difficulty in a role like this. In *Working together*, it says that the health authority should appoint a designated doctor, a designated midwife and a designated nurse to coordinate all aspects of child protection across the health district. But when you have separate trusts, that can present problems in terms of which organisation 'owns' those designated responsibilities." (designated nurse, case study site)[1]

Tensions over 'ownership' between the health authority and the trusts were manifested in the process of agreeing funding responsibilities for different aspects of the designated and named posts (such as providing training across the provider units). One named nurse argued that such disputes were becoming increasingly common:

> "... if you are looking at a post like a named health visitor which, prior to trust formation, wouldn't have been a matter of debate as to who

funded it, now there is much more demarcation between employers in terms of who should be doing what and who should be paying for it, and that even boils down to money split into directorates within the trusts." (named nurse, case study site)

The problem of funding responsibilities was exacerbated when the designated professionals were also responsible for the named roles. Staff in other agencies also reported concerns over the accountability of these positions. Thus non-NHS members of the ACPCs questioned whether designated health professionals had sufficient 'authority' or 'clout' with purchasers or providers, especially independent practitioners like GPs, to ensure that they recognised their child protection responsibilities. Problems were especially seen to result from the different lines of managerial and professional autonomy surrounding the designated/named staff and thus their ability to monitor the implementation of child protection policies and procedures across the service as a whole:

"Individuals within it [the NHS] are working more autonomously now and are not necessarily going to take notice of the procedures." (senior police officer, case study site)

Representation

Another issue arising from the purchaser/provider division in the NHS concerned the representation of designated and named roles on the ACPC and its sub-committees. A number of designated and named health professionals felt unclear about precisely 'who' they were representing – their own professional group, a particular sector of the service or the NHS as a whole. Other members of the ACPC, particularly those from outside the NHS, appeared to share this confusion:

"I think other professionals have some confusion, including health professions themselves when they're representing other disciplines. Quite often health representation will be from nursing, but they may be representing clinicians at the same time." (ACPC chair, case study site)

Most designated and named professionals expressed the view that first and foremost they saw themselves as serving the interests of a wide range of health practitioners rather than the health authority, or the more nebulous notion of the health service, per se. A few named professionals reported some tension between their involvement in direct operational matters and the more strategic concerns of the ACPC. This perception was articulated by one of the named nurses who had been delegated by a designated doctor to attend an ACPC sub-committee meeting:

> "... to be honest I didn't understand what on earth was going on. The things they were talking about didn't seem that applicable to the hospital, and I kept thinking what am I doing here? Am I the right person to be a representative of the health authority?" (named nurse, case study site)

Work coordination

Senior professionals from outside the NHS perceived that the greater diversification of service responsibilities within the NHS had made it more difficult for designated health professionals to ensure coordination of child protection practices and procedures across the health authority area:

> "If you wanted policies implemented you used to go to the health authority and they had their own lines of accountability and communication, but now you've got all these trusts. It's difficult for somebody from outside to get into these organisations." (NSPCC manager, case study site)

Interestingly, however, the designated and named health professionals themselves did not allude to this particular problem. Where difficulties around work coordination were mentioned, this was usually a reference to situations in which one health authority crossed over two local authority SSDs. This was true for the health authorities included in the study and was seen to introduce inconsistencies to child protection practice. For example, in one SSD it was routine practice to invite GPs to all child protection conferences, whereas in another adjacent authority there was more selectivity over the conferences to which GPs would be invited. Moreover, the amount of time needed to support two ACPCs had important workload implications for the designated members who also had a number of operational duties to fulfil. This was a particular problem for those who held the post on a part-time basis. Pressures of time were generally seen by designated doctors and nurses to limit their contribution to the development of a local interagency child protection strategy, at the very least by preventing them from attending all the relevant meetings.

Clarity over role

From the perspective of designated and named health professionals, one of the strongest constraints over effective role performance arose from the lack of clarity surrounding their professional remit. The 1991 *Working together* guidance recommended that the designated and named roles should be clarified in the contractual arrangements between the health authorities and trusts (Home Office et al, 1991). The relevant addendum (DoH, 1995b) stated that: "The role of designated doctors and nurses should be explicitly defined in their job descriptions and adequately resourced through the contracting process" (1995b, para 2.27, p 6). The findings from the Lupton et al study, however, suggest that, in practice, neither the definition nor the funding of the designated and named roles appears to have been adequately established.

The majority of designated health professionals were found to have written and developed their own job description *after* they had been appointed. Named professionals were less likely than their designated counterparts to have been given an explicit job description and revealed considerable diversity in the tasks they undertook. For example, two of the named doctors saw their role as mainly administrative while another was more clinically focused. Overall, the extent of involvement in the ACPC and/or its sub-committees was found to be extremely variable. Table 2 presents the self-perceptions of designated and named health professionals in respect of role clarity. While the majority of both designated and named professionals felt that role definition was adequate, this was truer of designated than named respondents. A sizeable minority of the latter (5 out of 12) felt that their role had not been adequately defined.

Table 2: Perceived adequacy of role definition and resourcing on the part of designated and named health professionals

	Designated [n=7]		Named [n=12]	
	Defined	**Resourced**	**Defined**	**Resourced**
Adequate	6	3	7	5
Not adequate	1	4	5	7

A few of the named professionals, particularly the nurses, felt that the lack of a well-defined role often led to the assumption by other health professionals that they were at their 'beck and call'. As one named nurse for accident and emergency services explained:

> "People see me as the person responsible for paediatrics, so they say, 'Here you are, you can deal with this'.... I don't have a clearly defined role in this department. I'm just seen as the person who deals with all the paediatric issues." (named nurse, case study site)

The sense of a certain devaluation of their role by medical colleagues was frequently articulated by the designated and named nurses who felt that doctors typically saw them as an additional pair of 'helping hands'. This was seen to be a result of the different power and status of the two professional groups, with doctors being more used to delegating to nurses than to consulting them on an equal basis. The poor uptake by hospital doctors and GPs of the child protection awareness training led by the nurse practitioners was also perceived to be due to the hierarchical nature of medicine and was considered likely to reduce the possibility of doctors participating in training run by nurses or, indeed, by non-NHS staff. Other nurse practitioners mentioned difficulties accessing information from clinicians:

> "... it's like walking through treacle sometimes because of professional boundaries." (named nurse, case study site)

Resource implications

Table 2 reveals that the (small) majority of both designated and named staff felt that the resourcing of their posts was inadequate. The lack of funding was seen to be reflected in issues of time allocation and workload manageability. Table 3 indicates the considerable variation in workloads, from under half a day for one designated doctor to between four and five days a week for other designated or named personnel. Many reported that their actual workload was greater than that suggested in the guidance (which appears to assume that additional responsibilities can be undertaken by senior doctors and nurses who continue to have full-time responsibilities in their main post) and that the time commitment the health authority was willing to fund for the child protection aspects of their post was

Table 3: Time allocated to child protection over an average working week as reported by designated and named health professionals

	Designated [n=7]	Named [n=12]
Less than a half day	2	0
1-2 days	1	5
3-4 days	0	0
4-5 days	2	1
variable	2	6

Table 4: Perceptions of manageability of child protection workload on the part of designated and named health professionals

	Designated [n=7]	Named [n=12]
Always	0	0
Usually	6	5
Sometimes	1	1
Rarely	0	6

inadequate. The exceptions to this were the designated nurse and named midwife in one case study site where, as part of a local initiative between the health authority and one of the SSDs, the two positions were funded on a full-time basis. Most other designated professionals felt that, while specific time had been allocated to participate in the ACPC and its sub-committees, other aspects of their post, such as providing advice, supervision or delivering training were not easily quantifiable and assumed a far greater time than was provided for in their contractual arrangements.

As Table 4 reveals, most designated professionals felt that their workload was 'usually' manageable but only because aspects of their main job and personal life were forfeited to make more time available for child protection work:

> "The time allocated isn't enough. I do the work that is required in the daylight at night-time; I do what hours I have to." (designated doctor, case study site)

Half of the named professionals said that they were 'rarely' able to manage the child protection aspects of their post and thereby were unable to 'do justice to the job'. While the commitment to child protection work among the named professionals was high, a number expressed flagging energy and enthusiasm for the post:

> "I have been told I can only do child protection for 15 hours a week, but you can't do child protection in 15 hours a week. If I decide that I am going to designate Thursdays and Fridays to child protection, then what happens on a Monday when a crisis happens?.... I don't hold out a great deal of hope of how it is going to work out." (named nurse, case study site)

Positive evaluation

The designated and named health professionals interviewed by Lupton and colleagues demonstrated a high level of personal commitment to their child protection responsibilities, with the designated professionals, in particular, emphasising their inclination and ability to take a stronger role in the development of local interagency child protection policy and practice. The desire to extend their role was not unrelated to their dissatisfaction with the lead role taken by SSDs:

> "I still feel uncomfortable with the 'ownership' of child protection by social services. I appreciate that they are the lead statutory agency but if you read the guidelines everything should be interagency, so I sometimes wonder if it's as interagency as it should be." (named midwife, case study site)

Non-NHS professionals appeared particularly to value the designated and named health professionals for their work in the provision of training and for their advisory and supportive role. Their impact on improving local health practice was seen to have been the greatest in hospitals and with the nursing profession and least in respect of general practice:

> "I think they are making an impact in hospital, they are making an impact with nurses. The big question mark on all of this are the GPs." (senior manager, SSD, quoted in Lupton et al, 1999b)

Table 5: Perceptions of regional ACPC members on the extent to which designated and named health professionals have improved the role of the NHS in local child protection networks (% of responses from NHS and non-NHS respondents)

	Designated professionals		Named professionals	
	NHS [n=52]	*non-NHS* [n=88]	*NHS* [n=52]	*non-NHS* [n=88]
To a great extent	15	13	10	15
To an extent	40	34	50	31
To only a limited extent	17	13	17	8
Not at all	8	3	13	5
Do not know	17	37	10	40
No response	3	–	–	1

This generally positive evaluation of the designated and named roles, however, contrasted with the findings of the regional survey of ACPC members undertaken by Lupton and colleagues. Here, views on the impact of the designated and named roles were mixed (see Table 5). Only a minority of NHS or non-NHS respondents felt that either of the two positions had improved the role of the NHS in child protection locally *to a great extent*. Exactly one quarter of health respondents felt that the designated posts had improved the health role either *to only a limited extent* or *not at all*. More respondents passed this verdict in respect of the named role. A minority of NHS respondents, and a much larger minority of non-NHS respondents, however, replied that they did not know what influence these key professionals had on the local role of health in child protection. Where explanations were given for this lack of knowledge, it was either because respondents were unaware of the existence of the post, or that the post(s) had only recently been created. At the time of the survey (completed at the end of 1998), one health authority appeared not to have appointed either a designated doctor or nurse.

Conclusion

We have argued that incumbents of the designated and named health roles have the potential to act as change agents in the child protection context. Primarily this is by contributing to the development of the cultural and technical infrastructure needed to integrate disparate health professional groups into the multiagency, interprofessional process of child protection. Designated and named professionals may thus play a central role in enhancing domain and ideological consensus within local provider networks. There is evidence to suggest, however, that despite high levels of personal and professional commitment on the part of those appointed, there are a number of factors impairing the effective performance of these roles. Unmanageable workloads, lack of appropriate post-qualifying child protection training, lack of role clarity and problems of representation and accountability are some of the main inhibiting factors emerging from the limited available evidence.

Any assessment of the change agent potential of the designated and named roles, however, needs to be taken in the context of the quasi-compulsory nature of the central guidance. The fact that this rests on the principle of 'you should' rather than 'you must' may account for the relatively slow pace at which health authorities and trusts have established designated and named posts. Evidence suggests that levels of funding and remuneration may also have inhibited the take-up of posts. Once established, there were indications that the effective performance of the designated and named role, especially by nurses, may have been undermined by tensions around professional power and status. Particular difficulties were experienced in respect of the responsiveness of GPs to the 'change agent' aspect of the roles. This reflects earlier research about the only limited involvement (or interest) of this group of health professional in child protection work (Simpson et al, 1994; Birchall with Hallett, 1995; Farmer and Owen, 1995). The next chapter focuses in greater depth on the role of the GP and the factors seen to limit their involvement in local interagency and multiprofessional networks.

Note

[1] All references from case study site are taken from Lupton et al, 1999b.

NINE

Sleeping partners: GPs and child protection

Introduction

General practitioners' (GPs') contribution to child protection is viewed as critical but the record of their performance is patchy. Research exploring the reasons for this suggests a number of factors are brought to bear, ranging from workload pressures and the inconvenient timing of meetings to some more fundamental concerns about GPs' perceived marginality of their role and issues relating to confidentiality. These rationalisations are worth exploring at greater depth, since they may also reflect the more fundamental dynamics of how GPs conceptualise their core role, and of the wider political agenda for general practice within the NHS.

While operating from a position of relative managerial autonomy, and therefore isolated from the regimes which increasingly govern the activities not only of the semi-professions but also hospital clinicians, GPs have been increasingly involved in service planning and exposed to the competing priorities of the health service. This chapter will argue that the low priority GPs currently accord to child protection work is an inevitable consequence of the profession's model of practice. It will also be argued that child protection's absence from current priorities for joint working between health and social care, and its resulting displacement to the periphery of health care 'business', have restricted the responsibility for child protection to a few, key personnel. In terms of Benson's model, there are insufficient 'resources' (money or authority) to attract the profession to participate in child protection networks as well as a number of 'superstructural dissonances' inhibiting collaboration.

The expectation and the record

The involvement of GPs in child protection processes is seen as essential, not only to the identification and referral of children but also to the process of determining an appropriate response to the situation. The *Working together* guidance (DoH et al, 1999) is quite firm in its conviction that GPs are centrally placed not only to identify children at risk of harm but to contribute to the child protection process at all stages. General practitioners are exhorted to provide relevant information to the child protection conference (CPC), whether or not they are able to attend personally. Despite the importance given to their role in a series of policy declarations (Home Office et al, 1991; DoH and Welsh Office, 1995; DoH, 1998b; DoH et al, 1999) and by other front-line workers (Simpson et al, 1994; Lupton et al, 1999b) research has raised questions about how adequately it is being discharged. Attendance by GPs at CPCs has been poor (Lea-Cox and Hall, 1991; Simpson et al, 1994) and GPs have been viewed as reluctant performers of their expected role by other participants in local child protection networks (Hallett, 1995; Lupton et al, 1999b; see Chapter Eleven of this book).

The reasons offered for GPs' limited contribution to the child protection process are various. One of the most important reasons cited for non-attendance was the timing and lack of notice of CPCs (Lea-Cox and Hall, 1991; Simpson et al, 1994; Lupton et al, 1999b). In Simpson et al's study, GPs who stated their satisfaction with the length of notice provided had a (mean) average notice period of 25 days. This may be realistic for GPs, given that surgeries, which may be timetabled two or three times each day, are often booked two or three weeks beforehand. General practitioners may also have other fixed duties, such as antenatal clinics, home visits or contracted sessions as clinical assistants. These are not responsibilities that can be easily delegated to partners, who have their own commitments. With time, GPs could arrange locum cover. However, the recommended fee for a minimum locum session of two hours is £83.50; currently GPs' reimbursement for attendance at CPCs of 1.5-2 hours is £60.20 (*MedEconomics*, June 2000). Thus there are seemingly perverse incentives in the arrangements for CPCs which appear to deter GP attendance. If GPs are not driven by economic motives alone (Hausman and Le Grand, 1999), however, other reasons may be needed to explain why they appear to prioritise the possibly routine medical needs of patients in a surgery session over those of children who may be at risk of abuse.

In addition to the inadequacy of notice, GPs have also indicated that the pressure of work in general compromises their ability to fulfil child protection responsibilities. Studies have reported a perception among GPs of a much-increased workload as a result of changes in the NHS.

These have tended to move the location of care from institutional to community settings, increased patient demands and generated additional bureaucracy (Hannay et al, 1992; Chambers and Belcher, 1993; Hiscock and Pearson, 1995; Scott and Wordsworth, 1998). Similarly, the involvement of GPs in fundholding and more recently PCGs/PCTs has extended their work to include service planning and development. These responsibilities and changed work requirements have coincided with a period of declining recruitment to general practice, possibly encouraging something of a 'siege mentality' among the profession.

In contrast to earlier research (Hallett, 1995), the majority of GPs interviewed by Lupton et al (1999) were clear about their role in child protection. However, some regarded their contribution as significant only at the pre-referral stage – before passing the case on to social services – rather than in subsequent arrangements (see also Moran-Ellis et al, 1993). This linear view of their role in the child protection process is confirmed by the perceptions of other front-line professionals in Lupton et al's (1999b) study who reported that GPs were seen to perform their role worse than any other professional group. It is difficult to say whether the GPs' views indicate a real ignorance of the role or a pragmatic accommodation, reflecting their perceived value to the process as well as other competing pressures on their time. There is evidence from a number of studies (Simpson et al, 1994; Birchall and Hallett, 1995; Lupton et al, 1999b) that GPs consider their contribution to the child protection process to be circumscribed. This may be partly due to the relatively low number of cases GPs see in comparison with 'specialist' workers. In one study, for example, GPs reported on average seeing fewer than two child protection cases per year (Lupton et al, 1999b) and, as a consequence, felt they had little experience in either the detection or management of child abuse. Yet, as Birchall and Hallett and point out, although GPs are frequently not well informed "… others who might expect to collaborate with them, had high, if unclear expectations of what [they] had to contribute" (1995, p 71).

In addition to their lack of experience in the child protection process, GPs indicated uncertainties over the diagnosis (sic) of child abuse, which were compounded by their limited contact with the families (Lupton et al, 1999b). Increasingly, the ways that GPs work – encouraging patients to attend surgeries, less 'ownership' of patient lists and the use of cooperatives or locums for on-call services – diminish the opportunities that they have to observe home conditions or develop detailed knowledge about families (Burton, 1996; Lupton et al, 1999b). The restricted nature of GP contact is evident in the fact that in 1991/92, 83% of consultations with the under-fives took place in the doctors' surgeries (RCGP, 2000). Furthermore, the gulf between others' expectations of GPs' ability to provide useful information and their own assessment of their contribution may act as an added deterrence to their attendance at CPCs.

The lack of confidence in themselves and the process expressed by some GPs is made more acute because of the perceived significance of referring a family to social workers. This act is seen by some as inexorably committing families to investigation and thereby criminalisation (Moran-Ellis et al, 1993; Lupton et al, 1999b). There are penalties enough if suspicions are confirmed, in terms of compromising relationships with patients, but a greater concern may be the additional harm caused by misdiagnosis (Lupton et al, 1999b). Some GPs in the study by Lupton et al felt that reliance on discretionary and sometimes intuitive judgements left them vulnerable to litigation. Certainly investigations of child abuse can traumatise those families involved and there are concerns among some GPs about their ability to deal with the emotions generated. Overlaying these anxieties is the duty medical practitioners have to keep information about their patients confidential, and this is discussed further below.

Histories, structures and cultures

There may be a number of relatively 'quick fix' solutions that could enable greater GP involvement in child protection, such as better notice of conferences and perhaps even locating these on GP premises, or encouraging more GPs to participate in child protection training. These remedies, however, skim the surface of what appear to be more deep-seated problems that deter GPs from engaging in child protection. Without first identifying and understanding these, more permanent solutions will be evasive.

While general practice attracts those who may be interested in a wide range of specialities it does not guarantee that all entrants to the profession will have a specific interest in child health. The *Framework for the assessment of children in need and their families* (DoH et al, 2000) calls for an understanding of the child's developmental needs as well as parenting capacity and wider family/environmental factors. Arguably prior knowledge in paediatrics would imply more of an interest in child health and surveillance, including the more specialised area of children in need, and would be likely to confer more confidence. In 1976 the Court Report (Court Committee, 1976) noted the fragility of primary care services for children within the generalist role of the GP and suggested the development of GP child specialists within practices. This proposal was dismissed by a profession that was not to be deflected in its struggle to establish the concept of the GP as a specialist in *general* and therefore comprehensive care.

Paediatrics is offered within the mandatory GP training schemes but the Royal College of General Practitioners (2000) noted with concern the difficulties of meeting the demand for posts offering suitable experience. More positively, however, recommendations for improved child health surveillance were endorsed in health service guidelines and the 1990 GP contract provided financial incentives to GPs' involvement in child surveillance. However successful, increased involvement in periodic examinations of the under-fives does not necessarily convert into a greater confidence in child protection matters, or a more specific interest in child health within general practice. Very few GPs according to one study, had volunteered for specific training in the handling of child abuse cases (Birchall, 1992). In the short term, developing an interest and confidence in child protection work may be a fortuitous consequence of the opportunities for closer working arrangements between GPs and health visitors that child health surveillance affords (see Butler, 1997).

Self-doubt about the value of their contribution, particularly in the post-referral phases of the process, may well reflect the changed nature of the child protection process and the reconfiguration of appropriate knowledge. The relatively recent history of child protection charts a progression from a dominant 'medical model' of child abuse, which characterised it as a disease best diagnosed and cured by medical professionals together with social workers, to one in which – following concerns raised in a series of child abuse inquiries – the judicial process dominated (Parton and Otway, 1995). Medical 'know-how' has become downgraded, both in child protection matters and more generally, a consequence of which is an increased sense of vulnerability in the profession. The primacy given to more intuitive, experiential forms of knowledge (see Chapter Three) is not only at odds with the epistemology of medical knowledge but also relies on exposure to a frequency of cases not apparently generated by the average GP list. In contrast, health visitors tend to cover several GP lists.

Although general practice may endorse the 'social' knowledge of individuals, families and, increasingly, communities, GPs are nevertheless trained to value what they see to be the *scientific* approach. This is critical of the validity of 'knowledge in practice' and encourages them only to disclose direct evidence of abuse in contrast with social workers who tend to assess risk on the basis of 'ecological' and circumstantial evidence (Sarangi, 1998). Furthermore, the scientific or evidence-based approach has been increasingly emphasised in the health service. Doctors, including GPs, are more frequently being challenged to justify their actions in terms of proven outcomes. This approach would find screening programmes that produce a large number of 'false positives' unacceptable, yet 75% of child protection referrals are dealt with before the conference stage (DoH, 1995b). While this is understandable given the rarity of definitive evidence and the ensuing vagueness surrounding the judgements, it may explain why some GPs regard their contribution as marginal to the process and, at best, 'diagnostic' only. Applying Benson's model, the possibly weak ideological consensus within the provider network over the identification and management of child protection cases may be sufficient to create 'disequilibrium' and compromise effective collaboration.

Although few GPs would dispute that the interests of the child are paramount, some are evidently reluctant to commit parents to a quasi-judicial process which appears to offer little therapeutic support for abusive families or for parents who lack adequate parenting skills. A referral may severely compromise the continuing relationships between the GP and the family. Though distant, the risk of complaint and possible litigation is of concern to GPs (Lupton et al, 1999b) who may be increasingly sensitised to this threat in the critical climate surrounding medical practice. For families the consequences are considerable. Included among the 'casualties' are those who receive a family visit during the early investigative stage but who are then eliminated from the system, stigmatised but not necessarily supported. Further along in the process, risk assessment continues to take precedence over therapy: "... too frequently, enquiries become investigations and, in over half of cases, families receive no services as the result of professionals' interest in their lives" (DoH, 1995b, p 39). Concerns about the adversarial nature of the process may encourage some GPs to distance themselves from it. This, paradoxically, may diminish their preparedness to support the child and parents and may place greater responsibility on social services and health visiting. On the other hand, the move to a 'lighter touch' and the shift from child protection to family support and children in need may, in so far as it emphasises the 'social' nature of the problem, also serve to distance clinicians who focus on their medical role.

The issue of medical confidentiality also remains an important one. This embraces relationships with the parents and possibly other family members, as well as the child. Concerns about the divulgence of sensitive information by medical personnel to social services has been noted in several studies (Simpson et al, 1994; Hallett, 1995; Lupton et al, 1999b). Although this fundamental ethic and legal duty is conditioned by a clear prior duty to act in the public interest, the uncertainty which may surround the early assessment of the situation – where vague suspicions are more in evidence than firm convictions – creates conflict and doubt. The DoH, in association with the BMA, produced guidance which observed, somewhat pointedly, that doctors may wish to test out initial concerns about child abuse before these "… are shared with non-medical colleagues" (DoH and Welsh Office, 1995, p 3) and encouraged doctors to discuss matters with senior or more experienced colleagues. Subsequently the definition was further clarified to involve "… a designated or named professional or a paediatrician or senior health visitor experienced in child protection" (DoH, 1996, p 13). Agency and, secondly, professional boundaries are clearly important in determining the propensity for sharing information, even where such information is encouraged to be anonymised (DoH, 1992b, p 4). It may be a tactical decision on the part of the DoH to encourage timely notification of at-risk children by keeping such preliminary discussions 'in house', but at a deeper level the guidance reflects the contested ownership of such knowledge, the authority and power associated with it and, adopting Benson's terms, the defence of a 'domain of high social importance'.

Interprofessional relationships are inevitably conditioned by the profession's collective view of the patient or client and the appropriate solution (Soothill et al, 1995), underpinned by different professional ideologies. Mention has been made already of the uncertainties surrounding referral which hint at distinctions between the biophysical, individual and curative focus of medicine and social work's concern with the social rehabilitation of individuals within families and communities. Although the intellectual leadership of general practice has promoted a more holistic, socially rooted, approach, Dalley (1991) still found distinct differences between the ideologies of social workers and health service professionals. These reinforced cultural divides between agencies and encouraged territoriality. Negative stereotyping of each other by health and social services professionals, one purpose of which is to cement and protect group solidarity (Dingwall, 1977, cited in Dalley, 1991), is evident in some accounts which examined child protection services (Birchall with Hallett, 1995; Hiscock and Pearson, 1995) and services more generally (Leedham and Wistow, 1992). However, a more recent study found little evidence of negative professional stereotyping of social workers by GPs, although frustration was expressed over different organisational cultures and the lack of feedback following referrals (Lupton et al, 1999b).

Closer working relationships with named social workers, including attachment to practices, have been proposed by GPs as a means of resolving process difficulties. These included both the damage done by triggering an inexorable process as well as, conversely, the reported reluctance of social services to respond with sufficient urgency (Lupton et al, 1999b; Moran-Ellis et al, 1993, Simpson et al, 1994). These contradictory criticisms suggest a lack of understanding by primary care team members of the thresholds of concern operating in child protection teams and of the way in which risks are assessed and priorities determined in order to rationalise the deployment of scarce resources. Although community care managers have been located in some practices (Leedham and Wistow, 1992), specialist social workers have not generally been so placed, presumably on the basis that time taken up by this level of liaison is better spent with clients. Both lack of confidence in GPs' ability to make a correct referral and reservations about social work practice are more likely to be remedied by more frequent and informal contacts. Furthermore, this arrangement may encourage reciprocity in the form of a more sustained involvement by the GP over the whole of the child protection process (DoH et al, 1999).

The discussion so far has identified some obstacles to GPs' greater involvement in child protection matters and has noted the relative low incidence of cases seen by some GPs, which contradicts some of the official optimism surrounding their significance in identifying cases. It has not, however, tackled the root question of why GPs choose to prioritise other work over child protection. As noted earlier, GPs view their workload as increasing inexorably and have been encouraged by the BMA to discriminate between core and non-core services (GMSC, 1996). The purpose of the guidance was to enable doctors to reject new work involving an extension of their services without payment. It is not suggested that child protection work would not be seen as a core service, defined elliptically as "... one which is normally provided by every GP" (1996, p 4) and as "... proactive services normally provided" (p 5). Interestingly, however, some categories of client groups familiar to social services were included in the non-core services section as were "... collaborative arrangements (eg with local authority social services departments or local education authorities)" (1996, p 6). This more market-oriented and discriminating approach to work may do little to encourage involvement by GPs in interagency work, such as child protection.

Applying Benson's theory, general practice may see little present resource value in claiming or maintaining what it instrumentally defines as 'peripheral' functions of the role.

Attempts at retrenchment on the part of general practice have to be evaluated within the wider context of developments within the NHS. These have reinforced the position of GPs and required them to participate in health service planning. Their new pre-eminence, however, has also reinforced their status and the unequal power they bring to local health care politics, including the micro-politics of interagency teamwork. Moreover, while some have enjoyed the new-found prestige and influence delivered by fundholding and then by PCGs or PCTs, others have regretted the incursion of managerial duties (Marks and Hunter, 1998; North et al, 1999). Rather than the pursuit of money or authority (as nominated by Benson), time has become the key desired 'resource'. Closer exposure to NHS managerialist principles which celebrate efficiencies, coupled with a greater emphasis placed on treatment in the primary care setting has, if anything, encouraged more delegation of duties to nursing staff, particularly practice nurses. The GP was traditionally seen as an autonomous and isolated professional, somewhat detached from the wider primary health care team and at the hinterland of joint social and community health care dealings. The primary care reforms have not reversed the independent nature of GPs' professional practice – surgeries and home visits are not team affairs. Neither have the traditional repertoires of general practice, which tend to be limited to relatively brief periods of contact before treatment or referral, been transformed. Nor has the status of GPs as the head of the PCT been displaced. Organisational changes may instead have encouraged the delegation of child protection responsibilities to health visitors or the mimicking of traditional medical practices whereby GPs 'refer on' to a specialist, who in child protection is the social worker. Such practices have not tended to facilitate effective teamwork within primary health care (West and Field, 1995).

The involvement of GPs in PCGs and PCTs, however, has inevitably meant that they have had to grapple with the strategic role of general practice and community health services in community care. Primary care groups are identified as 'pivotal' in the development of joint investment plans spanning the social/health care interface (NHS Executive, 1998). Such responsibilities, which will continue with GPs' involvement in PCTs, should at least mean that local leaders in general practice would become more experienced in interagency matters. The presence of the social services representative on PCGs is expected to improve joint working

(Secretary of State for Health, 1999) and the ADSS has set out an agenda which includes the development of operational links between social services staff, primary health care teams and GPs (ADSS, 1999). The prospects for improved understanding between GPs and social services personnel are better than at any other time in the history of the two agencies. Hudson (2000) suggests that SSD representatives on PCG boards, who have tended to be senior managers, are having an effect on commissioning and service delivery. A study by Glendinning and Coleman (2000), however, indicated that the perspective of SSDs carried less weight in PCG discussions than those of NHS stakeholder groups.

The prospects for child protection arrangements, however, are less clear. Although Glendinning and Coleman (2000) noted that there was convergence between the parties over the priorities for service development, these predictably reflected the traditional concerns of the health service. Only one third of social services appointees had any responsibilities for children's and family services, a position reflecting the pre-eminence of issues relating to other client groups on national and local agendas. The fact that child protection matters were not mentioned in the PCGs' priorities suggests the subject's low salience for the NHS or a reluctance on the part of social services representatives to raise potentially contentious issues at a time when the concern is to build relationships. Thus the involvement of local authority representatives on PCGs or PCTs may be circumscribed by agendas which are in turn dictated by the necessity of meeting the health needs of the local population. More broadly they are required to respond to the HImPs determined by health authorities in association with local authorities and other agencies. In the crowded agenda of PCGs/PCTs , the child protection process is only likely to merit special attention and effort if interest is signalled by the DoH or if events locally necessitate remedial action. The National Priorities Guidance 2000/01-2000/02 (www.doh.gov.uk/npg/), however, identifies other concerns for children's services.

A further difficulty relates to the *governability* of the wider GP constituency. General practitioner members of PCGs/PCTs have no formal authority over local practices, although they are authorised to make decisions about service developments on their behalf. This implies acceptance of the decisions made, but this is not modelled on the distant, representative democracy of Westminster. Important debates are likely to be aired in Local Medical Committee meetings, which all GPs are entitled to attend. General practitioner representatives on PCGs/PCTs may well be influential in directing discussions but they must remain loyal to the wider and possibly more conservative GP constituency. Their power over practice-level GPs is persuasive, not hierarchical. Any attempts at the PCG level to improve the contribution of GPs to the child protection process are therefore unlikely to be successful unless they are mandated by the wider group of GPs or manipulated through government incentives or sanctions. It is unlikely that GPs will support moves to encourage their greater participation unless the initiative reflects their preferences, for example, the allocation of a named social worker to liaise with practices.

The discussion thus returns to the issue of accountability (see Chapter Four) and to a central argument that, under the cloak of professional self-regulation, medicine has managed to avoid being held accountable for acts of omission as well as of commission. While the *Working together* guidance strongly suggests 'should' rather than requires the GP's involvement in child protection work (DoH et al, 1999, pp 19-20), there is an expectation that these duties will be fulfilled (see Chapter Six). Non-compliance with the guidance may leave GPs open to litigation, a threat which they are becoming increasingly aware of in other areas of work but apparently not in relation to their duty of care to children at risk of harm.

General practitioners are, in addition, more likely to be held to account by health authorities than previously. Although for the moment they retain the relationship of independent contractors, their activities have come under greater scrutiny. The rationale for the additional surveillance has been the necessity of demonstrating performance. This attracts payments rather than punishment, but has proved to be successful in modelling GP behaviour to support policy implementation. These incentives, coupled with the gradual absorption of GPs in strategic management, have inevitably broadened the scope of activities for which they can be held accountable. While measures that might reinforce the GP accountability in child protection processes are currently absent, the government's *NHS Plan* (DoH, 2000a) contains provision for the expansion of Personal Medical Services (PMS) contracts for GPs[1]. This will enable refinement in the contracting of GP services and could include, if the government so determined, a more robust prescription of the GPs' contribution to the child protection process.

Conclusion

In exploring the reasons why GPs have not been called to account for their lack of involvement in child protection work, we return to discussions concerning the relative autonomy of the medical profession compared with nursing and other semi-professions.

General practitioners, as with other groups within the health profession, have claimed autonomy as an essential precursor to serving the patient's needs. As a result, doctors have been able to organise and define the boundaries of their work, and that of the medical semi-professions, while being able to resist the application of bureaucratic rules to their practice. Instead, doctors have claimed the right of professional self-regulation through the offices of the General Medical Council and peer surveillance, mechanisms which have increasingly been found wanting. The professional autonomy enjoyed by GPs has been reinforced by their ability to avoid managerial surveillance. For many years the failure to integrate family practitioner services administration into mainstream NHS affairs, its capture by GPs with a collective reputation as idiosyncratic and unyielding, meant that their freedom was indulged. In relation to Benson's framework, GPs constitute a provider interest group powerful enough to control administrative arrangements and to shape the dominant policy paradigm in the health policy sector. However, there is some difficulty in situating GPs as an interest group within the more 'conglomerate' policy sector of child protection. General practitioners' power has been deployed negatively, to resist involvement in child protection processes. Perversely, this may be because the medical profession has been unable to dominate debates or, given the high level of state prescription, control the organisation of work. In addition, significant though its role is deemed to be, general practice gains few resources (in Benson's terms, income or authority) from its involvement in child protection, compared with those generated by its other responsibilities. Thus the profession can be seen to have largely excluded itself from participation in central or local child protection networks.

The situation may now be changing, with *The NHS Plan* representing a further step in the regulatory advance of the state. The difficulty remains, however, of monitoring a fragmented workforce and therefore of being able to call GPs to account for inadequate performance. The state's impotence in the past to ensure the accountability of the medical profession generally, and of GPs in particular, is, however, only a part of the answer. The de-prioritisation of child protection work by GPs is de facto condoned by both state and society. In recent years GPs have been positioned as 'informed' commissioners of local services. Given the considerable change agenda outlined for primary care, and the pivotal role sketched out for GPs, it is perhaps not surprising that successive governments have chosen to exercise their regulatory muscle on other matters. Undoubtedly children's services have been given additional impetus in central and local government with the multiagency approach of the DoH's Social Care Group and a more directive approach is discernable in initiatives such as *Quality Protects* (DoH, 1998c) and the 1999 *Working together* guidance (DoH et al, 1999). These nonetheless have competed for attention in an NHS which is concerned with seemingly more pressing issues of coordination between health and social care: the need to maintain those with long-term health and support problems in the community, and to restrict the use of in-patient care to those who are acutely ill.

Put more succinctly, the most significant stakeholder of all within the child protection sector, the state, has acquiesced in the present division of state-employed or state-contracted labour. Debates about these issues and the relative responsibilities of agencies are conspicuous at both national and local level, forming the principal landscape on which the dynamics of power between stakeholders are played out. The coordination of child protection, being the responsibility of SSDs, is less contested than the more ambiguous apportionment of resources in other areas. The more that GPs are absorbed into the local governance of the NHS, the more that their allegiance to health care as a priority is likely to be reinforced. Furthermore, until a critical mass of evidence materialises in which GP participation in child protection is found wanting, the profession's role may never occasion sufficient political resolve to challenge the status quo.

Superficially, there are a number of mechanisms by which GPs can be encouraged or required to contribute more to child protection. Professional peer pressure in support of clearly expressed standards may be the most effective in changing GPs' values. However, this remains an unlikely ideal given that the profession has not tended to value or prioritise its contribution to child protection work. What remain are sanctions – including the threat of litigation – and incentives. There are few incentives for GPs to report to or attend CPCs and no apparent sanctions sponsored by the NHS if they do not. Litigation currently seems a distant threat, given that GPs' distinctive contribution to the process may not be readily identified. The holding to account is therefore blurred by the difficulties of isolating the worth of the GPs' contribution and the derogatory impact on proceedings should they not participate. More thought needs to be given by government to closer regulation and encouragement of GPs' participation. Or, given the ambitious agenda already planned for GPs and the political energies required to redirect them towards participation in child protection, the government, as principal stakeholder, may be better advised to take the path of least opposition. In this context, a more radical option might be the formal delegation of child protection responsibilities to health visitors. This option, and the contrasting engagement of health visiting in child protection work, will be discussed in the next chapter.

Note

[1] In contrast to the national standard contract the PMS contract allows for a more discriminating approach, paying GPs on the basis of quality standards and negotiated targets based on local population needs. The new initiative, announced in *The NHS Plan* in July 2000, will see additional PMS contracts operational from April 2001.

TEN

Health visitors and child protection

The primary focus of health visitors' work with families is health promotion. Like few other professional groups, health visitors provide a universal service which, coupled with their knowledge of children and families and their expertise in assessing and monitoring child health and development, means they have an important role to play in all stages of family support and child protection. (DoH et al, 1999, section 3.35)

Introduction

As with other front-line professionals in health care, health visitors are viewed – and see themselves – as having a seminal role in both the identification of child protection cases and the subsequent management of cases. It is a role which, on a number of criteria, they appear to fulfil satisfactorily (Simpson et al, 1994; Birchall with Hallett, 1995; Lupton et al, 1999b), but which has also been subjected to constraints and tensions. These are derived from the changing political economy of health and primary care and concerns about the future of health visiting. They also reflect debates within the profession about professional–client relationships in the context of a process that has been dominated by judicial considerations and the determination of culpability. Following an account of the performance of health visiting in child protection, this chapter will deliberate the reasons for health visitors' commitment to child protection matters, whose record contrasts with that of their general practice colleagues. It will identify past and contemporary pressures faced by the profession in maintaining a multifaceted role. In doing so the chapter will explore current debates, which seek to resolve apparently dichotomous demands on the role, and will evaluate the profession's capacity to determine the future direction of the service and the allocation of scarce health visiting resources to child protection work.

An understanding of its history is helpful in contextualising current debates in the profession. Health visiting originated at a time when concerns about urban populations and the spread of disease encouraged the development of a public health movement. By the early 20th century, sanitary reforms had been completed and the state instead began to attend to individual and child health, an approach prompted by the poor physical condition of Boer War recruits. Advice and support for new mothers and the creation of child welfare services became the focus for health visitors' involvement. Within an overall responsibility to promote the health of the community, child health has been an ever-present and significant component. Since the development of community nurse attachment to general practice in the 1970s, the health visitor has worked alongside GPs, assuming the major part of the responsibility to routine child health surveillance.

The 1990 GP contract, however, offered financial rewards to those who became more involved in health screening for those children registered with them. For health visitors, this has meant a change in the way they operate, with more clinic-based attendance than formerly (Butler, 1997; Smith, 1998). Policy interest in child health is manifest in the Labour government's commitment to improving access to child health services as part of their strategy for the amelioration of social exclusion. The *Sure Start* scheme is integral to their overall strategy for greater inclusion of disadvantaged populations and has been largely welcomed despite unease over some faintly coercive elements (Hehir, 1998). However, while these new initiatives should assist in the surveillance of babies and young children, and are therefore not incompatible with child protection work, they also extend the responsibilities of health visitors to routine child health services.

The child protection role

Two complementary characteristics ensure the centrality of health visiting in child protection work: its universality, as recognised in *Working together*, and the fact that it is unsolicited (DoH, 1992b). Its universality means not only that case finding is likely to be more effective, a point not lost on the Court Report (Court Committee, 1976) or in central guidance on child protection, but also that the service is not associated with negative connotations of poor parenting and therefore does not stigmatise. The mandatory requirement that health visitors visit new babies at home in the first month, and may continue routinely to do so, does not excite public interest. Thus the universal nature of the service means that, for the most part, health visitors are welcomed or at least tolerated. Unlike GPs and social workers, health visitors are able to see the family home at least once and are more able to gain access subsequently without triggering rejection. However, the covert nature of screening for possible neglect or abuse, albeit a secondary agenda, has caused the profession some disquiet. There are ethical dilemmas in the role of the health visitor who gains entry to the home as adviser to and supporter of parents, but in effect acts as a covert observer for the state. Echoing the concerns of GPs over medical confidentiality and their longer-term relationships with families, Taylor and Tilley (1989) argue that a statutory duty to disclose information would clarify misconceptions. This, however, does not circumvent ambiguities about the health visitor's role with those parents whose child has been placed on the child protection register.

Historically, work with young children and their families has formed the greater part of the health visitor's working day (Dunnell and Dobbs, 1982; Brown 1997). Unsurprisingly, both the *Working together* guidance and the views of other key workers in child protection recognise the essential contribution of health visiting. In Simpson et al's (1994) study, social workers rated the attendance of health visitors at Child Protection Conferences (CPCs) as more essential than that of GPs. Similarly, in comparison with the roles of other health professionals in child protection, the role of the health visitor was regarded as paramount by 81% of NHS front-line respondents and 70% of non-health front-line respondents in the study by Lupton et al (1999b). These views also embrace performance. Despite concerns noted earlier, health visiting appears to have fully embraced its responsibilities in child protection. Health visitors were found to have participated in over 81% of case conferences in Simpson's study and in Lupton et al's study the majority reported that they had attended all the CPCs to which they had been invited in the previous year. The research further reported that at least one health visitor attended each of the sample of 120 CPCs observed during the fieldwork.

Beyond attendance, health visitors appear to be functioning effectively in other aspects of the child protection role: 95% of health and 93% of non-health respondents in Lupton et al's (1999b) study judged them to have performed their role well. Health visitors in another study were also regarded as being 'very' or 'fairly' easy to work with and their performance was rated positively or very positively by over 94% of the other respondents (Hallett and Birchall, 1992).

The contrast with research evidence on the contribution of GPs and, to a lesser degree, other health professionals, such as accident and emergency clinicians and paediatricians, could not be more stark. This raises the question of why health visitors comply with and perhaps exceed the baseline requirements of official guidance in relation to their role, while GPs tend to underperform. Some explanations are superficial. Although health visitors would argue that they are as equally hard-pressed as their medical colleagues, their work routines probably allow more flexibility than those of GPs to accommodate short-notice CPCs. However, if the sentiments expressed and the volume of literature devoted to child protection are an indication, health visiting also seems to accord a greater salience to the subject and to the contribution it makes, than does the medical profession. The centrality to health visiting of child health work and child protection matters is evident. In determining why this is so, this chapter will locate its explanations within the broader context of health service reforms and the politics of the profession. In so far as the contribution of the agency (for example, the community trust) is, to a large degree, synonymised by health visiting, these issues will be discussed in relation to Benson's 'interorganisational' framework (1975, 1983).

Health visiting's determination – as a part of a professionalising project in common with other branches of nursing – to demonstrate high standards of performance no doubt plays a part. In parallel with this is the need to define and safeguard an area of professional practice that is discrete from, or in some way superior to, the expertise of other professions. Child health surveillance and community health promotion have traditionally been claimed as health visiting's professional territory, but the rapid development of practice nursing has presented something of a threat to health visiting's health promotion role (McDonald et al, 1997). The balance of resources allocated to the two key responsibilities has been variable and locally conditioned, and is particularly contentious in contemporary debates about the future of the profession. Health visiting's motivation to maintain its role in child health surveillance is a necessary but insufficient explanation for the high level of involvement in child protection work. There are extrinsic compulsions also. The compliance of health visiting with official guidelines reflects its status as a semi-profession operating within the state's regulatory capacity and its place within a professional and team hierarchy. In the hypothetical and unlikely situation that the profession de-prioritised child protection duties, it could not easily evade them. Neither would it be able to delegate responsibilities to GPs, the other members of primary health care teams with a significant contribution to make.

While not wishing to repeat the debates in Chapter Four, it is worth emphasising the point that health visiting, like nursing, has never operated independently of either local authority or health service administrations. Unlike the medical profession, which before the NHS largely operated a fee for service arrangement[1] and so maintained its independence via the professional–client relationship, the state was the employer of health visitors. The latter thus had less opportunity to market their skills to the private patient than did midwives or nurses. Until the 1974 reorganisation shuffled district nursing and health visiting into the NHS and rudimentary primary health care teams, health visiting was a part of the Medical Officer of Health's empire. Doctors were also pre-eminent in the NHS. As major stakeholders, medical professionals had been able to secure influence in decision making at all levels of the health service, as well as considerable autonomy in professional practice. Although the practice/domiciliary locale of the work and a much flatter hierarchy meant that health visiting was less open to scrutiny than hospital nursing, the former has been as much defined by the requirements of health authorities, and latterly trusts, as by the profession. The firm guidelines handed down to local health authorities, such as *Working together* and its sequels, reflect a bureaucratic process, and the manner in which compliance is secured is essentially hierarchical in nature. Health visitors, like social workers and police officers, have little discretion in the matter. They are accountable to their employers as well as their profession. Unlike GPs, they have less room for manoeuvre and the consequences of non-performance of their role in child protection are more obvious – because they, in effect, delegate for absent GPs. The reverse situation does not obtain, the differential status of health visiting and medicine, and the reluctance of the former to bend practice guidelines, being a possible explanation for their acquiescence in this arrangement.

The above discussion may appear somewhat theoretical, since health visitors have willingly embraced their responsibilities in child protection, but it is important as a counterpoint to the body of evidence emphasising the internalisation of standards. A frequent theme in the literature emphasises the need to establish and maintain optimal performance in professional tasks (Warner, 1993; Goodwin, 1994). Normative claims reflect the need to safeguard standards but also convey to onlookers the image of health visiting practice operating at a 'professional' standard. As such, they should be contextualised in health visiting's long and determined claim for professional recognition. Child protection is no different from the other functions of health visiting, the exception being that failure may have spectacular and deleterious consequences for the profession as a whole. This is further reinforced by the fact that, second only to social workers, the occupation is viewed as being most closely identified with child protection work and therefore more culpable than most if things go awry. The costs associated with failure are therefore high, making it all the more necessary that child protection work is work well done and in compliance with official guidelines.

A part of the task of the successful profession is the establishment and maintenance of control over a professional territory. Ironically, health visiting's drive for professionalisation has entailed delineating and justifying a professional identity separate from nursing. Other community nurses may be involved in children's *nursing*, and therefore potentially the identification of child protection cases. Health visiting, however, because of its statutory role in health surveillance, has secured a professional niche that sets it apart from nursing. The threat to the health visitor's professional territory from medicine has been more oblique, resulting from the financial encouragement of GPs to become more involved in child health surveillance. The consequence of this for health visitors has been a loss in autonomy. In one study, health visitors felt there was an unnecessary duplication of roles. Home visits had been reduced and community clinics disappeared to be replaced by practice-based surveillance clinics (Butler, 1997). As a result of the new payments for GPs for child surveillance, health visitors' work became more visible and its execution more central to the business that is general practice. This did not necessarily extend to child protection, where the contribution of the medical profession has become more marginal. Since the downgrading of medical knowledge in the 'diagnosis and treatment' of child abuse (see Chapter Three), GPs have become less dominant as experts. Moreover, circumstantial evidence suggests that, while GPs may view child protection as intrinsically important, it does not take priority over their other duties, which they are contractually and professionally obliged to fulfil. Health visitors are regarded by some GPs as the child protection 'expert' within the primary health care team (Simpson et al, 1994; Lupton et al, 1999b). Nor can gender be ignored in GPs' relationships with a profession that, more so than nursing, has been a predominantly female one. Society expects that women undertake the care of the vulnerable and the child in need of protection is one of the most vulnerable members of society. Nevertheless, while GPs have supported health visitors' pre-eminence in the role, changes in general practice have eroded the ability of health visiting to execute it effectively.

We have argued that, in health visiting, 'boundary maintenance' has been necessary to safeguard child surveillance and the place of child protection work. This does not apply in relation to social work where organisational considerations of resource protection take precedence over professional concerns. In Benson's terms there exists a firm *ideological consensus* between health visiting (and by extension community trusts) and social workers (qua SSDs). The goal is not so much to promote health visiting's involvement in child protection as to define and limit its contribution so that it can develop other professional roles. The investigation and coordination of child protection matters, in accordance with statute and firm guidelines, are unequivocally the responsibilities of SSDs. The problem for the health visitor is to manage the scope of her involvement so that an appropriate balance is achieved between the relatively peripheral though important responsibilities of child protection and the bread and butter work of child health surveillance and, increasingly, community health. Issues of *domain consensus* which may affect interorganisational relationships between SSDs and community trusts are therefore more likely to be concerned with defining and limiting involvement – which for the organisation will protect expenditure and for the profession will preserve time and energy to address other territorial matters.

The need to secure a place for health visiting in the new public health movement will be discussed below; however, the tensions within health visiting are not simply between family-centred child health surveillance (and by default child protection) and community health promotion. Within the nature of child protection work the changing emphasis between family control and family support presents opportunities as well as difficulties. The broader role promotes health visitor involvement but, as noted earlier, there is some discomfiture with, though recognition of the necessity of, the involvement of the disciplinary state in the protection of vulnerable children. The more preventative approach endorsed in the 1999 *Working together* guidance is broadly welcomed by the profession. For health visiting, however, the difference in emphasis may exacerbate the difficulties already experienced in relation to thresholds of concern and the need to involve social services' personnel in cases well before formal referral takes place (McDonald et al, 1997; Lupton et al, 1998).

This more proactive approach may pose a greater difficulty for the profession, that of role overlap with social workers. There is a danger that health visiting will be increasingly drawn into the task of supporting vulnerable families in place of social work. This scenario is made more likely by the broader health-associated concerns generated by the new public health movement and by health visiting's traditional focus on poverty and inequality. The most immediate risk is that, in the overall organisation of child protection, health visitors become more conspicuous members of a team managed by social workers. While this may more comfortably fit with current policy approaches endorsing interagency collaboration, it has consequences for professional autonomy and may also compromise health visiting's current professional project, which is to secure its claim to community health work.

Organisational change and professional politics

The maintenance and furtherance of health visiting's professional autonomy has been a long-standing objective, in keeping with the strategies of other professions. This professionalising project not only saw a challenge to medicine's definition of nursing (and health visiting) knowledge but also to medicine's right to control what nurses do (Witz, 1992). Health visiting, more so than nursing, has succeeded in developing a body of knowledge and a therapeutic direction independent of mainstream medicine – although not of the new public health medicine. It was an intellectual trajectory that also successfully translated into a degree of organisational independence. Along with midwives, health visitors were the least well integrated into the primary health care team (Wiles and Robison, 1994). Where teams operated, they were often dominated by GPs but the peripheral situation of health visitors, combined with the introspective gaze of general practice in the 1970s and 1980s, created a directional void which permitted health visiting to operate with some autonomy. The Griffiths management reforms (see Chapters Four and Five) from 1984 onwards strengthened bureaucratic control of health visiting. However, the lack of engagement with the initiative by hospital and community clinicians, coupled with the fact that general practice remained something of a hostile frontier for NHS management, enabled health visiting to retain some independence from medical control.

General practice fundholding threatened this arrangement. GP fundholders were able to renegotiate the detail, if not the broad principles of, community nursing contracts. This gave them considerable leverage over other members of the primary health care team. The sudden relocation of power, away from neutral management to the profession that represented the greatest threat to health visiting autonomy, was unpalatable. It was not, however, strong enough to threaten, in Benson's terminology, the equilibrium of the interorganisational child protection network. In general terms, the change to GP purchasing did not present a challenge to health visiting's involvement in child protection per se, since GP fundholders were required to conform to health authority advice and ensure that child protection was a 'key component' (DoH, 1996, section 2.25) in contracts. However, the leverage that contracting gave to GP fundholders, and GP commissioning groups more generally (Moon and North, 2000), coupled with the inducements in the new GP contract to undertake child health surveillance, had an important influence on health visiting practice. Health visitors in one study felt that they had lost control over the prioritisation of their work, that there was duplication of surveillance work between GPs and health visitors and that the internal market in general had led to a reduction in resources for community child health (Butler, 1997). The result was that home visits were curtailed as child health surveillance was increasingly undertaken in GP surgeries. These issues were echoed in a Health Visitors' Association survey that showed widespread concern over the demands of the contracting process. It was felt that this had concentrated resources at management level (child protection officers) as well as creating a 'perverse incentive' for clinic as opposed to home-based visits (Leach, 1997).

The internal market brought health visitors under the contractual leverage of GPs, thereby compromising the wider aim of nursing – and by default health visitors – to shake off medical control. The 'elevation' of GPs to fundholding status arguably presented more of a conceptual challenge to the autonomy and status of health visiting – since nursing has claimed a parity with medicine as a profession – than the ability of purchasers to engineer extensive changes in the way that health visitors operated. The change in status, however, proved the less durable problem. GP fundholding disappeared in 1998 but the pressure on resources and the need to demonstrate effectiveness persisted. Vestiges of the purchaser–provider split remain inherent in present arrangements, whereby primary care groups/trusts (PCGs/PCTs) have taken over the majority of purchasing responsibilities from health authorities and the disbanded fundholders. Nevertheless, the creation of PCGs provides an opportunity for health visiting and social services to have a voice in the development of local services and to reinforce the importance of children's health services and, in principle, child protection. Potentially, this may enhance the work coordination dimension of Benson's interorganisational equilibrium.

The emphasis on cooperation within the health service (DoH, 1997) has signified a return to a more collegiate approach among health professionals which in turn has strengthened the hand of community nursing. For the first time since the consensus management of the 1970s, nursing has been included in the planning of health services. At face value the arrangements for PCGs/PCTs suggest a more pluralistic approach, with local authority and lay representation on boards. Applying policy network theory to the local level, this may appear to constitute an issue network in the local governance of the NHS. Interim research on 12 case study PCGs (Smith, 2000) suggests that the district nurses and health visitors who made up the nursing membership of the 12 PCGs saw it as an opportunity to present a nursing perspective in decisions. In a survey, which unfortunately did not solicit the views of GP members, they were rated as the fourth most influential members (after chief executive, chair and GPs). However, the qualitative responses indicated a less assured role. Stakeholders in five PCGs commented on the exclusivity of the process and the dominance of GP members. Tellingly, respondents felt that the chair and chief executive collectively made the most significant decisions in PCGs. All chairs are GPs. This may not engender the collegiality desired in policy statements.

One conflict of interest may relate to pressures to contract for services that demonstrate their cost effectiveness. This is also likely to be an imperative for the PCTs, which are destined to supersede PCGs. As Goodwin (1994) noted, community nursing outcomes are more difficult to define (and evaluate) than more general clinical outcomes, because success is less tangible. In the case of child protection, positive outcomes relate to the prevention of acts, which are difficult to discern, or to the timely identification of dysfunctional or 'dangerous' parenting. The preference of health visiting for home visiting is likely to be countered by the pressure on other PCG board members to secure cost-effective services. It is also likely to be resisted by the interests of GPs, which lie in the location of health visiting resources in practice-based clinics rather than home-based child surveillance. Pressure to change services to conform to these ideals may not be easily countered by the nurse and social work representatives.

These issues are part of wider tensions between the NHS and social care in which responsibilities for elements in the welfare of a number of client groups are ill-defined and subject to debate. In this, child protection work is less ambiguous than, say, elderly care, as the guidance produced by the core policy community is more specific about roles and responsibilities. However, this level of specificity does not extend to the manner in which professional roles are executed, nor does it commend a minimum standard in relation to the amount of health visiting resource devoted to children's health and development. Benson is not silent on these matters (1975, 1983). The dynamics of an interorganisational network are conditioned by external factors such as new administrative arrangements. The greater responsiveness of the public sector to the state's demands and the requirement that they operate 'Best Value' services, represent new rules of the game which create the context in which local provider networks operate.

Debates about the best, most cost-effective, use of health visiting skills at the local level are reflected in deliberations within the profession over the most appropriate way forward. As we have indicated, the health visitor's professional role is greater than child health surveillance, which generates its involvement in child protection work. Health visiting has retained, from its earliest days, responsibility for health education and promotion although in many areas this aspect of the role has been more muted. The development of a 'new' public health, involving a community focused and integrated approach requiring the cooperative efforts of a number of local agencies, has provided an opportunity for health visiting. Its role in health education was noted in *The health of the nation* (DoH, 1992c), in the Labour government's White Paper on public health (DoH, 1999b) and has been most recently signalled in the White Paper on the contribution of nursing, *Making a difference* (DoH, 2000c). Although these and other policy initiatives indicate a number of strands in health promotion, ranging from individual advice to community development, there has been particular interest and investment in community-wide approaches. Although the literature reflects evidence of health visiting's engagement with community development work, however, this aspect of health visiting lies "... outside mainstream health visiting practice, and [is] largely unrecognized" (Craig and Smith, 1998, p 176).

The profession is therefore presented with something of a dilemma. It has been confronted with a number of opportunities or demands, the development of which may compromise its success in other areas. Like any other profession, there is a concern to consolidate, as well as advance, professional territory and this encompasses community approaches to health as well as, at the other end of the scale, individual health and well-being. There is currently much discussion in health visiting literature of the relative merits of these claims (Twinn, 1993; Craig and Smith, 1998; Carnell et al, 1999). The difficulty for those who seek to promote its involvement in community health work is that health visiting is already stretched by its commitments to new babies and their families. Despite elaborate models of public health practice, which incorporate both child health surveillance work and holistic approaches to community health promotion (see Carnell et al, 1999), the reality is probably fettered by the restrictions of caseloads and requirements placed on health visiting services by PCTs and health authorities. Thus the debate returns, in circular fashion, to local 'voices' in health visiting on PCGs and PCTs, as well as those of its national leadership.

Conclusion

It is the 'elasticity' of health visiting's role that presents problems as well as opportunities for the profession and this, coupled with the need to secure its own interests, has produced a period of uncertainty and internal debate. The Community Practitioner and Health Visitors' Association, which symbolically extended its name from the Health Visitors' Association, is in the process of developing a model of practice which incorporates individual, family and community levels of action (Carnell et al, 1999). It is a matter of some doubt whether individual health visitors can accommodate a more ambitious public health role – one that in effect requires a community development agenda – as well as maintaining their family caseloads. A more logical strategy may be to create the public health specialist within the profession. Having exhorted health visitors to develop their public health role with families and communities (DoH, 1999b), government policy gives little direction on the pressing question of how local resources will be marshalled to support the more demanding duties.

Much then may depend on the local politics of commissioning. It is unlikely, given the firm guidance of the central policy community (DoH, 1996), that health visiting's commitment to child protection work will be deflected into other activities. Thus, whatever the postures of the constituent members of the interorganisational child protection network, their operation is constrained by firm parameters dictated by the state. Indeed, in recognition of recent patterns of GPs' and health visitors' respective contributions to the post-identification phase of child protection work, a more sensible approach might be to designate the health visitor as the primary health care team's representative and key worker in the child protection process. This would clarify responsibilities and legitimise the role that, de facto, many health visitors assume. Arguably, until this formalisation of current practice takes place, health visiting will not be able to claim more resources. Nor will it have the capability to develop the otherwise welcomed recent 1999 *Working together* guidance, which asks all participating agencies to "... consider the wider needs of children and families ... whether or not concerns about abuse and/or neglect are substantiated" (DoH et al, 1999, section 2.26). As we write, it is a critical time for health visiting and for its role in the child protection process. Specialisation within the profession may be the only means of securing high standards of practice, either in family caseload or community health, in the future.

Note

[1] This statement holds true at a general level, although the majority of GPs also had a 'panel' of patients who paid National Insurance sickness contributions and received, in turn, medical care and medicines when sick.

'Healthy' networks? NHS professionals in the child protection front line

Introduction

This chapter concludes our examination of the operation of provider networks in child protection. Its aim is to illuminate the experience of collaboration on the part of the main health professional groups engaged in child protection work at the front-line level. Studies of interprofessional and multiagency cooperation have tended to stress notions of 'reciprocity' and 'consensus' and have typically under-emphasised the factors that may operate to impair effective collaboration. One reason for this relative inattention to conflict is the way in which the network is conceptualised. Approached metaphorically, the idea of 'networks' suggests an interconnected web of well-established relationships, "... a smoothly interlocking system of reciprocal roles" (Whittington, 1983, p 268). The focus of analysis is thus typically on the composition or structure of this relationship system. Attention to the *dynamics* of interprofessional networking, however, rather than to their formal structure, is also important and may reveal a number of underlying conflicts or tensions. As much as the conditions of reciprocity, the areas of tension may be instructive in explicating the day-to-day operation of a particular network.

To understand these dynamics we have argued the relevance of Benson's (1975, 1983) model of the 'interorganisational' network as a mini 'political economy' (a series of mutual resource dependencies) operating within a wider political economy (the relevant policy sub-sector/sector). Within networks, effective collaboration will hinge on the degree of equilibrium obtained across four dimensions (ideological consensus, domain consensus, positive evaluation and work coordination). Factors both internal and external to the network, however, may operate to disturb this equilibrium on any or all of its key dimensions. These may be the result of sub-structural elements (wider organisational/professional imperatives) affecting the internal balance of power and authority. Or they may be external, resulting from the links of member groups/organisations to power relations within the wider policy sector or society more generally. For Benson, three possible states of disequilibrium may follow:

- *forced coordination* (high on work cooperation, but low on domain or ideological consensus and positive evaluation);
- *consensual inefficiency* (low levels of work coordination, but strong on domain and ideological consensus and positive evaluation);
- *evaluative imbalance* (high on work cooperation and strong on domain and ideological consensus, but low on mutual positive evaluation).

It is useful to add to this typology the theoretical possibility of other ideal–typical states:

- high positive evaluation, but low ideological and domain consensus and weak work coordination (*evaluative inefficiency*);
- high levels of ideological and domain consensus, but poor work coordination;
- negative evaluation (*forced consensus*).

Particularly in networks characterised by multiprofessional as well as multiagency participation, it is also possible that there may be situations characterised by agreement regarding the role of each agency (strong domain consensus), but disagreement in respect of the nature of the tasks faced and the most appropriate way of achieving these (weak ideological consensus), and vice versa: strong ideological but weak domain consensus. Following the Benson schema, we would label these states as respectively, *domain inefficiency* and *ideological inefficiency*.

This chapter sets out to apply the Benson framework to the specific context of child protection provider networks. The degree of consensus which can be seen to exist across each of the specified dimensions is examined and the specific contribution of health professionals and agencies to the achievement (or not) of network equilibrium is assessed. In the context of the limited evidence on the contemporary role of health professionals in child protection work, the chapter will draw extensively on the findings of a large-scale empirical study carried out by the authors at the end of the 1990s. The particular elements of this wide-ranging study of relevance here are the questionnaires completed by front-line health (n=48) and non-health (n=127) professionals in the three case study sites and the in-depth interviews undertaken with GPs (n=100) in two health authority areas (see Introduction for more details).

'Healthy' or 'unhealthy' networks?

Collaboration does not occur automatically. As Whittington (1983) argues, effective collaboration between disparate groups or individuals should be seen as an 'accomplishment' that is achieved through a series of negotiations or bargains around particular courses of action. Bargains do not, however, take place on a level playing field. Perceived or ascribed differences in power and status between professionals, their different levels of skill, knowledge and access to resources, means that certain groups will have more influence over the terms and outcomes of collaboration than others. In particular, much will depend on where individual members are 'positioned' within the network – how centrally involved they are in its actions and agendas. Described by Hallett and Birchall as "... ever-changing coalitions among a large number of professionals in different locations and groups" (1992, p 232), the local child protection networks are characterised by variable levels and frequency of engagement on the part of those who can loosely be defined as 'members'. Using Webb's (1991) typology of intensity of involvement, it is clear that the relationship between some participants approximate the 'routinised' end of the continuum, with close and regular contact providing the opportunity to develop understanding and appreciation of each other's roles and responsibilities, to bridge ideological differences and effectively to coordinate work. In contrast, other situations of interprofessional interaction in child protection may more closely resemble the 'radical' end of the continuum, characterised by limited and irregular contact and more likely to involve misunderstanding, imperfect communication and low levels of mutual evaluation.

The *Working together* guidance recommends that interagency/professional cooperation should cover all stages of a 'case career', from the initial referral stage through to registration/de-registration. The evidence suggests, however, that few professional groups other than social workers are involved in all stages of the process and that various types of professional interactions are found, from fleeting exchanges to ongoing sustained joint work (Hallett, 1995; DoH, 1995b; Hallett and Birchall, 1992; Lupton et al, 1999b). Birchall and Hallett's (1995) study revealed a local child protection network operating on four interacting layers: social workers, the police and paediatricians at the central 'core' layer; health visitors, teachers, GPs at the second 'generic' layer; lawyers, accident and emergency staff and psychiatrists at the third 'case specific' level; and professional groups such as school nurses, education welfare officers and youth workers at the final 'peripheral' level.

The situation identified in the locality studied by Hallett and Birchall, however, may not reflect the picture nationally where there is evidence of considerable variation in the nature of the front-line network. Thus Lupton et al (1999b) found that it was health visitors, rather than paediatricians, who were involved in the sort of sustained joint work (high rates of attendance at CPCs and routine involvement in the management of individual cases) that would be expected of a 'core' professional group. They also found that, in one locality, school nurses were as highly involved in child protection as health visitors. School nurses, however, rarely figure in the literature on child protection, affected possibly by the narrow stereotype that links them to head lice and school medicals. In yet another locality, Lupton et al found that a 'core group' made up of two social workers, an education welfare officer, a specialist police officer and a health visitor functioned as a local strategic forum. Unconnected to the ACPC, this group oversaw the management of all child protection cases covered by local social work area offices. Again, whereas probation officers were identified in Hallett and Birchall's investigation as having a fairly peripheral role in child protection, Lupton and colleagues found their level of involvement in child protection cases to be relatively high.

Domain consensus

It is clearly important for the effective operation (equilibrium) of a network that its different participants are clear about the roles and responsibilities to be performed by themselves and other members. This may be particularly so for networks, such as those in child protection, that are involved in service provision. In their review of 32 child abuse inquiry reports, Reder et al (1993) found that role confusion or duplication, resulting from ambiguity about professional tasks, was a key factor in eight of the cases. Lack of role clarity on the part of professional participants has been highlighted in many empirical studies of local child protection networks (Stevenson, 1989; Blyth and Milner, 1990; Hallett, 1995). Lupton et al's more recent study (1999b) suggests that the situation remains uneven.

The majority of NHS respondents reported being either 'very clear' or 'fairly clear' about the role of their own professional group. There was greater variation, however, in their understanding of the roles of other health professionals. From a list that included health visitors, GPs, paediatricians, psychiatrists, school nurses and accident and emergency nurses and doctors, NHS staff appeared to be clearest about the role of the health visitor and least clear about the contribution of accident and emergency doctors. In respect of non-NHS participants in the network, health professionals were most certain about the role played by the social worker but much less certain about those played by criminal justice agencies such as the police and probation. For their part, non-health professionals reported that, in respect of the NHS contribution, they were clearest about the roles of the health visitor and the school nurse and least clear about the roles played by paediatricians and accident and emergency doctors:

> "Social workers and health visitors work closely with schools for the good of the child involved. School nurses too. Police and doctors tend to be quite distant figures in my experience." (head teacher, front-line questionnaire)

One finding from the Lupton et al study, however, was that, while NHS staff were generally clear on their own roles in child protection, there was evident a (large minority) perception that many *other* health professional groups lacked clarity about their roles in child protection. This was a charge that was particularly, although not solely, directed at medical professionals:

> "I am sure of the role they should have, but GPs and A&E staff seem to have little or no comprehension of child protection roles, situations or issues." (health visitor, front-line questionnaire)

For their part, however, the paediatricians and the GPs interviewed claimed to be generally clear about their respective roles in child protection and felt that the problem lay in the lack of clarity, particularly on the part of non-NHS staff, about the differences between health disciplines:

> "Sometimes social services don't understand differences in the role between a paediatrician and a police surgeon. If you need to get a child examined, a paediatrician is very well qualified to do it, but in a

child protection point of view it has to be a police surgeon, and police surgeons aren't employed as consultants in hospitals as such, they are freelance and we have to trawl them in and they are not there on tap. It's very easy to say, 'But you have all these doctors in your trust, what are they doing?' but only two happen to be police surgeons. If you go to a paediatrician he is perfectly well qualified to examine the child and come up with a diagnosis, but if you took that to court, it would get thrown out.... So there is a lack of understanding." (designated doctor interview)

The other area of disparity in terms of mutual clarity of roles occurred between social workers and health visitors. Whereas most social work respondents reported to be clear about the role of health visitors, the latter considered that many social workers were actually not very clear about the health visiting role, often either under-utilising their knowledge and skill base and/or expecting them to undertake tasks more appropriately performed by social services:

"People don't often realise our level of training or our amount of input to families. We are often just seen as people who just weigh and measure, which is totally inaccurate. I often feel my opinion is less valued particularly by social workers." (health visitor, front-line questionnaire)

Positive evaluation

In Hallett's (1995) study, apart from the social worker, the most 'essential' professional groups identified by network respondents were paediatricians and specialist child protection police officers. These were followed by accident and emergency doctors and then health visitors. This order, Hallett suggests, reflects the dominance of investigation within the child protection process. Lupton et al (1999b), however, found that, while both health and non-health professionals saw the role of the social worker as the most essential, it was the health visitor who was generally seen to be the next most important, perceived to be playing a more 'essential' role in child protection than either the police or paediatricians. The performance of health visitors in the detection and interagency management of child abuse was highly rated by both health and non-health respondents alike. Social workers, in particular, reported a high level of input from health visitors in child protection and considered that they were one of the easiest professional groups with which to work.

In general, NHS respondents tended to rate the importance of other health professional roles more highly than did their non-health colleagues. The majority of non-health respondents felt that GPs, paediatricians and accident and emergency staff were 'important' rather than 'essential'. They also assigned greater importance to the school nurse role than did their NHS colleagues, with teachers especially valuing the nurse liaison with SSDs. Despite the GP being seen as either 'essential' or 'important' to child protection work by the great majority of both health and non-health professionals, Lupton et al's study confirms previous findings of widespread dissatisfaction over the role of GPs in child protection (for example, Lea-Cox and Hall, 1991; Simpson et al, 1994; Hallett, 1995). General practitioners were identified as the professional group performing least well in the child protection process by NHS and non-NHS respondents alike. Only accident and emergency doctors were rated less positively overall. It should, however, be noted that many respondents (health and non-health) felt insufficiently informed to evaluate the role of accident and emergency staff in child protection, a finding which, in itself, suggests a fairly marginal role for these staff in local child provider networks. In addition, medical professionals were generally viewed by both nursing practitioners and non-health professionals as the most difficult professional groups with which to work in child protection:

> "GPs are often difficult, unable to comprehend the broader issues and seem frustrated at having to attend case conferences." (social worker, front-line questionnaire)

The relatively poorly perceived performance of medical professionals was felt by many health and non-health staff alike to derive from their reluctance to accept their child protection responsibilities. The lack of attendance by doctors at CPCs, for example, was often seen as an indication of the low priority they accorded to child protection work:

> "GPs and A&E staff do not behave as if they are part of *Working together*." (health visitor, front-line questionnaire)

Health visitors generally tended to be more critical of their health colleagues, particularly GPs, than did professionals outside the NHS. Indeed, the study appeared to uncover some fairly deep tensions between health visitors and GPs, with the former expressing resentment at what they felt was a case of the latter's 'passing the buck' for child protection work on to them:

> "GPs are often only interested in what is profitable. I don't think they want to deal with these difficult families and issues." (health visitor, front-line questionnaire)

Doctors and hospital-based health professionals were seen by many other network participants to 'position' themselves in the interagency process of child protection in a very distinctive way. Their perception of interprofessional working, it was felt, was of a process in which each professional contributes in succession, in a division of labour, or 'chain of care'. Many doctors were seen to perceive their role as limited to the early identification and referral stage, typically involving little more than the exchange of information with other child protection professionals. This approach was felt to contrast strongly with the more team-based approach of other health and non-health participants in the network:

> "We all have time restraints and increasing demands, and the absence or failure of GPs to contribute to a conference is frequently felt to be an indicator of their unwillingness to be involved as part of an interagency approach to working with children and their families." (social worker, front-line questionnaire)

The evidence from GPs themselves appears generally to confirm the view of others that they see their child protection contribution as limited to the initial identification and referral stages:

> "Once the initial information is gathered, thereafter comes the management, the safeguard of the child. The help tends to come from people other than me. I need to be kept informed, but I don't really have a direct input into the therapeutic side of things." (GP interview)

This position was due not only to GPs' perception of their role as appropriately diagnostic, but also to the changing nature of general practice. The impact of the changes in the GP role, it was widely felt by GPs, had not been fully appreciated by child protection professionals:

> "I think to assume that GPs are front-line identifiers [of child abuse] is

a sign of the lack of knowledge of the way GPs work these days. We're not in the homes seeing everything.... We see people in surgeries for 10 minutes when people come to us with a problem." (GP interview)

Accident and emergency health professionals similarly felt that most agencies and professionals, including the primary health care team, had unrealistic expectations of their role in child protection work. Workload pressures, ambiguous physical signs and the lack of wider information on the child and family, were seen to limit the role these staff could play in identification:

"Children always fall over and bump their head, bump their knees, whatever, and that's how children present, with very plausible injuries and explanations. How we are supposed to identify those that aren't [accidental] isn't always easy. Say a child comes in with cigarette burns, bite marks, anyone can spot that. But the vast majority of our children don't present like that. We don't have the information on the family background that they have. I don't know that there's an easy solution for that. If we see a child who provides an easy, plausible explanation for an injury, we have to take it from that." (accident and emergency nurse, front-line questionnaire)

Other constraints over a more extensive input on their part that were articulated by GPs and hospital doctors were the lack of child protection training, anxiety over making a wrong diagnosis and/or fear of making matters worse by notifying social services:

"... [there is] a lack of personal responsibility to take this forward. The orthopaedic surgeons don't want to know, so they don't deal with it, as they don't like it. Everyone's frightened of it. They're concerned with the implications...." (named doctor, strategic interview)

Concerns about confidentiality were widely identified as creating difficulties for medics in sharing patient information with other agencies. Non-health colleagues tended not to be too empathetic with these concerns, however. Social workers and police officers in particular tended to feel that the issue of confidentiality was a way for some practitioners to avoid involvement in a case or to 'sit on the fence', particularly if involvement required attending court to give evidence. Whatever the reality of the situation, it was clear from this study that a major feature of the front-line networks was the dissonance some health professionals experienced between the way they saw their roles and the way in which others perceived those roles. Different expectations of roles and responsibilities is a major factor in domain disequilibrium and may also serve adversely to lower the level of positive evaluation that exists between network participants.

Ideological consensus

There is evidence from the Lupton et al's study that, in many cases, tensions surrounding domain consensus were exacerbated by different professional approaches and frames of reference about the cause of child abuse and how it should be addressed (ideological consensus). On the one hand, there was evidence of the tension between the traditional preventative and curative role of the nursing professions and what was seen to be the more investigative role of the child protection social workers and the police ("We have officers who come charging in to wards which isn't particularly helpful. Softly, softly, is a lot better" – midwife, front-line questionnaire). General practitioners in particular expressed concerns about what they saw to be a hasty and over-zealous response on the part of social workers ("I mean, sometimes the actual abuse may not be as bad as the consequences of informing social services" – GP interview). On the other hand, there was also evident a contrasting view of social workers, held by some health visitors and their medical colleagues alike, as being too slow to act due to much lower thresholds of intervention ("We tend to want to get in there early on. I guess social workers see that sort of thing all the time and are more tolerant" – health visitor, front-line questionnaire).

In general, opposing views about the nature of the problem and the appropriate action to be taken were identified by around 3 out of every 10 respondents as 'sometimes' causing conflict between front-line staff:

> "It's bad enough trying to come to agreed plans about what to do when we are clear that abuse has taken place, but it starts to get really tricky in cases of neglect and emotional abuse which are more difficult to define. What health sees as important isn't necessarily what others see as important." (health visitor manager, strategic interview)

There was also evidence, particularly on the part of hospital-based paediatricians and accident and emergency doctors, of disengagement from what were seen to be the more 'social' dimensions of child abuse, in respect of which they felt they had little or nothing to contribute:

> "There are many situations in which we don't have a role. We don't have anything to contribute medically, so it isn't an issue for us." (GP interview, case study site)

'Social' in this context was defined in terms of the wider family situation and the influence of factors such as poverty and deprivation on child neglect and abuse. In this way, the broader child welfare approaches of health visitors and social workers were contrasted with the more clinically focused concerns of doctors. This demarcation was also related to perceived differences in the 'core business' of health and SSDs:

> "We've identified the areas where we badly differ, so at least we know where the sticking points are, and one of those sticking points is our complaint that we cannot get post-abuse treatment because it's not prioritised in child and adolescent mental health. 'Abuse' is seen as a social issue and not a medical one." (senior manager, SSD, strategic interview)

Important differences were discernible among health professionals, and between NHS and non-NHS colleagues, about the role of the central *Working together* guidance and local practice protocols. Considerably more importance was attached by health visitors, along with social workers and the police, to compliance with central or local guidelines than was the case with the medical professionals. Concern was expressed by the nursing professions and the community-based paediatricians about what was seen to be an over-emphasis on the potentially punitive process of investigation at the expense of more supportive, preventative measures. The main area of resistance to central or local practice guidance, however, came from medical professionals. Many GPs and hospital doctors perceived the current guidelines to be too rigid and argued for greater flexibility to allow for professional autonomy and discretion:

> "The guidelines are useful as a framework, but you've really got to be a lot more flexible, and I think the essence of good child protection is networking and really getting to know who's who, on a very basic level really, and cut through a lot of the so-called procedures." (hospital paediatrician, interview, case study site)

As with confidentiality, however, the doctors' appeal to 'clinical freedom' was met by other professional groups with a degree of suspicion. For some it was felt to be used advantageously by doctors to maintain their professional autonomy and thereby enable them to stand 'outside' the rules that applied to everyone else. Underpinning these attitudes were seen to be issues of power and status. Perceived differences in professional power were particularly expressed about GPs and hospital doctors, and largely, but not solely, by health visitors and social workers ("The paediatricians tend to talk over every one's heads" – social worker, front-line questionnaire). In particular, tensions around the sharing of information were seen to be linked to issues of power and status ("Power and confidentiality. These to me are linked, because the confidentiality reason can be used as a power badge by certain professionals" – health visitor, front-line questionnaire). There was some reciprocal disparaging of social workers' skills and experience, mainly by GPs ("Social workers tend to have less experience than their age suggests" – GP, interview), but generally the study found relatively low levels of the disciplinary hostility or stereotyping reported in other studies of interprofessional collaboration (Broussine et al, 1988; Leedham and Wistow, 1992). By and large, judgements about the performance of other professionals appeared to be taken on an individual basis ("... [it] varies according to the individual and the team" – GP, interview). The major area of concern about the contribution of other professionals groups derived not from judgements about their professional experience, but from differences in the ways in which their working day is organised.

Work coordination

A major problem identified in the Lupton et al study was the practical difficulties of establishing effective communication and coordination between agencies with very different forms of work organisation. These proved to be obstinate barriers to the coordination of child protection activities and to the pooling of knowledge. Thus, a common reason advanced by GPs for not attending CPCs was the logistical problem of their working day being structured tightly around surgeries (see Chapter Nine). Other professionals, such as teachers with classroom timetables or consultant paediatricians with scheduled clinics, also appeared to experience similar constraints. The frustration this caused for other professional groups was clearly evident:

"I find it difficult to get information from A&E doctors.... It's hard to track people down on different shifts, and often doctors working on the night shift don't pass on information to daytime staff. This makes it difficult for police and social workers to get a full picture of events." (police officer, front-line questionnaire)

These differences, however, were not just between professionals working in different agencies but also between professionals working within the NHS. From the perspective of accident and emergency staff, for example, it was the absence of formal channels of communication between their departments and the primary and community services that left them feeling organisationally and professionally 'isolated':

"As a department it feels very much like operating in isolation, we don't have sort of very routine links with GPs, surgeries, health visitors, social workers, whatever." (accident and emergency nurse, front-line questionnaire)

Communication difficulties were seen to have increased with the diversification of service providers within the NHS and their different lines of managerial accountability. The main problem expressed by those outside the service was knowing precisely with whom cooperation needed to take place:

"My experience with dealing with health is that it is very difficult to know who the right person is in terms of getting them to conferences, and knowing who the right person is in terms of who holds the purse string." (social worker, front-line questionnaire)

Lupton et al found that the recent experience of local government reorganisation had also impacted on work coordination. The reorganisation and relocation of social services offices was reported to have created difficulties in knowing where to send referrals and was felt by many to have disrupted local child protection networks cultivated over the years ("the people changed, faces changed" – health visitor, front-line questionnaire). Hospital-based health professionals, in contrast, tended to report that levels of communication and personal contact with social workers had greatly improved following local government reorganisation. In one hospital at least, this had resulted in the establishment of a dedicated paediatric social work team.

Conclusion

The available evidence suggests marked variations in the roles played by different health professional groups at the individual case level. Although the situation is likely to differ between localities, investigation across three case sites (Lupton et al, 1999b) indicates a high level of involvement and interest in child protection matters from health visitors and paediatricians and, in one area at least, from school nurses. This can be contrasted with a generally low level of engagement in child protection from GPs and accident and emergency doctors, particularly following identification. One main reason for this variability is the different levels of 'exposure' to child protection and thus the less 'routine' nature of interagency collaboration experienced by some professional groups. Certain health professionals, such as midwives and health visitors, have an opportunity to observe the daily interactions of the family unit and, as a result, are more likely to come into contact with child protection issues. Others, such as GPs, have much less scope to interact with young families than is perhaps assumed by fellow professionals or, indeed, within the *Working together* guidance (Lupton et al, 2000). The low involvement of GPs in the planned multidisciplinary intervention process needs to be understood in the context not only of working arrangements which afford them little time to engage in ongoing child protection work, but also their inexperience of (and possibly disinclination for) multidisciplinary ways of working. For accident and emergency doctors and nurses, the high turnover of both staff and patients, their relative isolation from primary and community health services and their lack of information on the family background, are all factors reported to limit their contribution to child protection work.

To an extent, the evidence suggests a reasonable degree of *domain consensus* surrounding the roles of specific professional groups in child protection. Most appear clear about their own role and that of other key players in the process. One of the most important findings in the Lupton et al study, however, was a mismatch between the expected (or perceived) roles of certain professionals and the actual roles being performed. General practitioners and accident and emergency professionals, in particular, indicated that their child protection role is often less significant than assumed by others. Differences between professional groups over expectations surrounding certain professional roles, results in role confusion and, if certain professional roles are not performed the expected way, to low levels of *positive evaluation*.

Even when certain professional groups demonstrate a high level of engagement in child protection work, however, and follow roles according to the 'script' (in terms of the roles outlined in the *Working together* guidance), barriers to collaborative working may persist. Increasing workload and time pressures are highlighted in the data as factors impairing the ability of professionals to contribute effectively to sustained multidisciplinary child protection work. These and other organisational differences limit the achievement of effective *work coordination*. The data also confirms that the ability to work cooperatively can be constrained by existing power relations. Groups with greater professional status may ignore, or be indifferent to, the efforts of other 'less' powerful occupational groups to maximise joint benefits through collaboration. Perceived differences in professional status were among the difficulties reported by some social workers and nurse practitioners in securing cooperation from doctors in respect of child protection concerns. The findings from the Lupton et al study also highlight ongoing tensions as a result of very real differences in professional cultures and approaches, adversely affecting *ideological consensus* about the nature of the tasks faced and the most appropriate way of achieving them.

The quality of interprofessional relationships in child protection also appears to be affected by wider changes at the central policy level. There is evidence that the diversification of service providers within health and local government reorganisation has created or increased difficulties of cross-agency/professional communication, impacting on *work coordination*. At another level the available data suggest that changes in the way child abuse is conceptualised – notably the shift in the late 1980s from identifying and treating *child abuse* to a concern with *child protection* – have significantly affected interprofessional relations. Most health professionals tend to see themselves at either the diagnostic or the 'caring' end of child protection, rather than the investigative part of the process. NHS professionals also diverge in respect of their interest in the broader child welfare arena. Those with a wider child health remit, such as health visitors, school nurses and, to a lesser extent, community-based paediatricians, were more likely to assume responsibility for family support and prevention than were groups like GPs and hospital-based professionals.

The evidence suggests that the child protection front-line/provider network may be too fluid to fit precisely into any ideal–typical model of network equilibrium. While the degree of *domain consensus* is relatively high (not least as a result of the *Working together* guidance), there is evidence of divergence in terms of expected and actual roles, in respect of some professional groups. The achievement of both *ideological consensus* and *work coordination* appears uneven, with the former impaired by disciplinary and status differences and the latter adversely affected by more practical organisational differences, especially in respect of work arrangements. In so far as these differences result in perceptions of lack of commitment to interagency child protection work, they may serve to undermine the extent of *positive evaluation* between certain professional groups. In terms of the ideal–typical models set out in the Introduction, the evidence suggests that the operation of child protection networks most closely approximates that of *domain inefficiency:* reasonable levels of domain consensus, but limited ideological consensus and work coordination and uneven positive evaluation.

Importantly, however, the discussions presented in this and earlier chapters also suggest that administrative fiat alone is clearly not sufficient to bring about reciprocal, mutually supportive actions on the part of groups with diverse interests and approaches. The impact of the coordination mandate at the local level may be undermined by the assumption not only that professionals have the appropriate skills and knowledge to work together to protect children, and possess sufficient understanding of, and respect for, each other's contribution to do so effectively, but that they are willing to collaborate in order to share a common burden of responsibility.

TWELVE

Conclusion

Since the original decision to keep the NHS organisationally distinct from the other aspects of the welfare state, improved collaboration between health and social care services has been a major policy objective. With the 'hollowing out' of the state and the emergence of a more 'differentiated polity' generally, and with the creation of internal markets within public sector services more specifically, the need for 'cross-cutting' solutions to enduring social problems became more acute. By the same token, however, the achievement of those solutions may be commensurately more difficult. On a practical level, public sector fragmentation increases the number and type of agencies involved and thus the potential for organisational or disciplinary dissonance in joint work. On a deeper level, there may be tensions between the exhortations to collaborate and the competitive ethos of the marketplace. The separation between politics and administration, moreover, and the growth of 'intermediate agencies' may make it less easy for the central state to provide effective overall coordination. As the 20th century drew to a close, there was a growing concern on the part of the international policy community about the discord between the precepts of new public managerialism (NPM) and the principles of good governance (World Development Report, 1997).

The search for ways to improve collaboration between the NHS and social care services has been most active in respect of community care, but has also characterised the development of services for children and their families. Particular pressures for greater collaboration in child protection resulted from a series of official inquiries highlighting poor liaison between different agencies and professional groups. Effective collaboration may be especially difficult to achieve in the child protection context, however, as a result of the sheer number of different professions and agencies involved. The NHS may experience particular problems in respect of collaborative work, given its complex organisational structure and its diverse professional groups.

The historical response of governments to the lack of collaboration has been to develop new mechanisms and procedures to underpin joint work. In child protection, these have ranged from the establishment of

Area Review Committees (ARCs) (now the ACPCs), joint child abuse registers and interdisciplinary case conferences, to the detailed prescriptions of the *Working together* guidance and the incorporation of child protection work into wider national performance and assessment frameworks. Together these mechanisms can be seen to represent the attempt by central government to 'mandate' the coordination of agencies and professionals at a local level (Hallett, 1995). The gap between policy objectives and their implementation, however, is as enduring a policy problem as poor agency collaboration. The central aim of this book has thus been two-fold: to assess the nature of the 'mandated cooperation' of the child protection process and to identify those factors that may undermine its achievement at a local level.

The changes in the organisation of the state during the 1980s and 1990s saw increased prominence given to the idea of 'policy networks' as a way of understanding the policy-making process. Developed most extensively in the UK by Marsh and Rhodes (Marsh and Rhodes, 1992; Rhodes, 1997; Marsh, 1998), this approach sees networks as structures of resource dependency, differentiated from both 'hierarchies' and 'markets'. Typologies of network theory provide a continuum from the small, consensual and tight-knit *policy community* (or 'iron triangle'), involved in frequent and high-quality interaction, to the looser-limbed, more unpredictable *issue network*, engaging less frequently and with less consensus. A key issue for empirical application of the network approach is the extent to which policy making in specific areas can be seen to have moved from the dominance of 'iron triangles' to the emergence of more diffuse issue networks.

As indicated, however, the core focus of this text is on the nature of the gap between policy ambitions and policy outcomes and this highlights the relationship between those making policy at a national level (the policy community) and those involved in its implementation at local levels (provider networks). The policy network framework proved to be of only limited use in understanding the nature of this relationship or for exploring the dynamics of front-line provider or 'delivery networks'. The text thus also utilised the interorganisational analysis developed by Benson (1975, 1983) in the US to assess the relationships between these networks and the central policy community. Benson hypothesises that effective interorganisational networks will achieve equilibrium across the key dimensions of *domain consensus* (who does what), *ideological consensus* (how it is done), *positive evaluation* (how well it is seen to be done) and *work coordination* (the practical arrangements for doing it). This equilibrium, however, is affected by the imperatives that constrain participant agencies as a result of their operation within the wider 'political economy' of the public sector. These imperatives relate centrally to the need to ensure a secure supply of resources (money and authority), to defend specific organisational (and professional) paradigms, to maintain public support and legitimisation and to pursue distinctive service objectives. In turn, these factors are underpinned by the power relations that characterise the wider policy sector and society more generally.

The national policy community

Applying one of the typologies of network theory (Wilkes and Wright, 1987), child protection policy can be seen as a specific dimension of the broader 'children and families' section of the 'social care' sub-sector of the generic policy area of 'health'. Health policy making has been presented as a classic example of the dominance of the traditional 'iron triangle' of ministers, civil servants and medical professions (Richardson and Jordan, 1979; Haywood and Hunter, 1982). Despite some inroads to the 'producer capture' of the policy process over the late 1970s and in the 1980s, medicine has largely retained its central place in health policy making, albeit at the price of succumbing to greater political scrutiny and firmer self-supervision. The health policy sector, however, is not homogeneous. Even within a particular sub-sector such as 'social care' there are many policy divisions whose characteristics may differ from those of the core health policy community. Within these, the role played by specific health professionals, and the NHS more generally, is likely to vary.

Although its configuration is difficult to map precisely, the national child protection policy network appears to involve a small tight-knit core, characteristic of the 'policy community' end of Marsh and Rhodes' continuum (Marsh and Rhodes, 1992; Marsh, 1998). Centred on the DoH, this core group also involves the (albeit irregular) participation of other key government departments. This interdepartmental configuration means that collaboration may be less 'routinised' than in the ideal-typical policy community, involving a potentially less cohesive form of 'radical' collaboration: the "... crossing of boundaries between mutually exclusive, competitive, or previously unrelated interests and domains" (Webb, 1991, p 231). This central policy community can be seen to operate within a wider issue network. Although more diverse and less consensual than the central policy community, this issue network is nevertheless more stable and predictable than any ad hoc collection of 'interested parties'. The relative strength and stability of its relationship with the core policy community suggests that the most appropriate metaphor for the child protection policy 'architecture' is that of a policy network with core and peripheral layers.

However, the relationship between the 'core' and 'periphery' of the national child protection policy network is uneven. On the one hand, it is characterised by a broad degree of consensus between the two layers, not least as a result of the high political visibility and sensitivity of child protection policy. The appearance of cohesion, moreover, is maintained by the declared determination of the core group to base decisions on widespread consultation and research-based evidence. On the other hand, the sensitivity of the child protection issue also necessitates close central political control of decision making, with the consultative process largely focusing on fine-tuning the broad policy decisions made by core decision makers. As Haywood and Hunter (1982) argued in respect of other areas of NHS policy formation:"... iron triangles may be less exclusive because some policies are processed in an extended range of groups [but] a closed system can still operate" (1982, p 161). The core group is by definition exclusive and tensions between it and those not directly involved in substantive decision making may never be far from the surface.

The local provider networks

In addition to the national policy community and issue network, child protection involves multiagency and interprofessional networks operating at the local level. These provider or 'delivery' networks comprise two main tiers, the 'case-specific' joint working of front-line professionals and the more 'strategic' collaboration of agency/professional representatives within the ACPCs. The ever-more inclusive remit of legislation and guidance means that, at both these levels, the child protection service is characterised by the involvement of a wide range of health professionals. Within the NHS, these may be drawn from both primary care (for example, health visitors, GPs, community paediatricians, dentists, school nurses, police surgeons, midwives) and secondary care sectors (for example, accident and emergency staff, hospital-based paediatricians, obstetric, gynaecological and genito-urinary staff). Considerably more is known about the child protection roles played by some health professionals than others, however. Although the *Working together* guidance briefly outlines their anticipated contribution, very little is known about the actual nature of the role played in local child protection networks by, for example, dentists, mental health services staff and hospital-based paediatricians. More evidence is required on the contribution of these professionals and, in particular, on the extent to which they have received "... the training and supervision needed to recognise and act upon child welfare concerns" recommended in the 1999 guidance (DoH et al, 1999, p 23).

The available evidence suggests that the involvement of different health professional groups in local child protection networks is uneven. At the front line, for example, the relatively high level of engagement on the part of health visitors and community paediatricians can be contrasted with the low or irregular participation of professionals such as GPs and accident and emergency staff. However, the evidence also suggests that the participation of different health professionals varies between localities. Thus, one study (Hallett, 1995) positioned the paediatrician, with the police and social workers in the 'core' layer of the network, and health visitors, with GPs and midwives, in the next, 'front-line' layer. Another (Lupton et al, 1999b), however, found the role of the health visitor to be central to the local network, across all stages of a case 'career', and that of the paediatrician and the midwife to be fairly marginal. This study also revealed the contribution of the school nurse (relatively unexamined in the literature) to be nearly as central as that of the health visitor. All available evidence, however, confirms that the involvement of GPs in the child protection network is extremely low (Hallett, 1995; Simpson et al, 1994; Moran-Ellis et al, 1993; Lupton et al, 1999).

Participation within the ACPCs by health professionals and/or managers appears to be extensive and greater, in volume at least, than representatives from SSDs and the police combined (Sanders et al, 1997). Again, however, the evidence suggests considerable variation from one locality to another. A key issue for local ACPCs appears to be achieving the right balance between sufficient NHS representation to cover all the main aspects of a highly fragmented service on the one hand, and protecting against the numerical domination of health members on the other. As with front-line work, involvement in ACPCs is variable on the part of different health groups. Professionals such as community nurses, health visitors and midwives play a greater role than groups such as paediatricians, child psychiatrists or officers from health authorities/trusts. Again, as with front-line work, the lowest overall level of involvement, relative to their centrality in government guidance, comes from GPs.

The creation of 'designated' and 'named' child protection posts (doctors and nurses) within the NHS was designed to improve the contribution of health professionals at both front-line and ACPC levels. In particular these staff have the potential to act as 'change agents', working to improve knowledge and practice across the different organisational and professional domains of the NHS and with those outside the service. The available information on the operation of these specialist posts, however, many of which are undertaken on a part-time basis, suggests that their impact may be limited. Despite the considerable personal skills and enthusiasm of incumbents, their contribution is typically constrained by heavy workloads, limited relevant experience, uncertainty surrounding their precise responsibilities and lack of appropriate training.

The strategic network

The role of the ACPC is central to the 'mandated coordination' of child protection networks, providing an essential bridge between the policy objectives of the central community and the operation of front-line services: a "system within a system" (Sanders, 1999, p 264). Successive versions of the *Working together* guidance have sought to enhance the role of the ACPC and to align its operation more closely with centrally devised performance management and assessment frameworks. There is evidence, however, that the capacity of the ACPC effectively to discharge its coordinating role may be restricted by its lack of statutory status and by the only limited ability of many of its members to effect operational change within their organisations. Central to the constraints surrounding the work of the ACPC are issues of accountability, representation and governance.

Different agency and professional participants within the ACPC will be subject to different configurations, or points of 'balance', between managerial, democratic and professional forms of accountability. To the extent that they represent contrasting expectations and priorities, the different 'accountability profiles' of constituent agencies/professional groups may undermine the equilibrium of the ACPC network. At best they may introduce creative tensions within the ACPC, with the development of more genuinely cross-cutting approaches to joint working. At worst, they could undermine the ability of the ACPC to reach consensus on key aspects of local practice or to operationalise any decisions made.

While all ACPC members may experience some difficulty in this respect, the organisational diversity of the NHS may make its role particularly problematic. Thus, for example, the (largely) successful resistance of the medical profession to the rise of the managers means it is less susceptible than other professionals in child protection to central regulation and control. Tensions between managerial and professional lines of accountability may thus lead key health professionals to assert their independence from priorities or procedures agreed (or unresisted) by those within other member organisations. At the same time, despite the rhetoric of devolution, the lack of democratic accountability within the NHS may mean that both managerial and professional staff are less accountable to local communities or electorates than many of their ACPC counterparts.

More prosaically, the issue of representation is potentially difficult for NHS staff as a result of the complex organisational structure of what can only very loosely be called 'a service'. Although the NHS is not unique in this respect, with many other public services experiencing increased organisational differentiation over the last two decades, its historically more fractured nature and the greater extent of its purchaser/provider divide, may make for particular difficulties. Many NHS participants in interagency forums, for example, may experience confusion about whether they are representing their own professional sub-group, health professionals more generally, a particular sector of the service, or even some general sense of the NHS as a whole. Even those managers with arguably a clearer representational brief may only be able to reflect the interests, and deliver the cooperation, of a very limited part of the service. Although established in part as a response to this situation, the role of the designated health professional serves to encapsulate the difficulties involved. Funded by the health authority, but employed by provider trusts, many designated staff are unclear precisely which side of the service they are representing or to which they are accountable. The reality of this tension is underlined by demarcation disputes between purchasers and providers about the responsibility for funding different aspects of the designated and named posts.

Given the above, many NHS members of ACPCs may find it difficult to adopt the role of representative *of*, rather than simply being *from*, a particular discipline or service sector. While it is possible to an extent for members who are trust and authority managers to provide some form of corporate capacity, this is much less the case for nursing and clinical staff, especially for autonomous practitioners such as GPs. Even those with a general service remit, however, may be limited in the extent to which they can commit their organisations to a certain course of action, particularly if that action carries resource implications. Again, this difficulty is not restricted to NHS managers, being shared with other services, such as education, which have devolved decision-making structures. It is the combination of many different types of accountability and governance that makes this problem particularly acute within the NHS.

The assumption of the *Working together* guidance is that better cooperation of senior agency/professional staff within the ACPC will make for improved collaboration at the operational level. There is evidence, however, that the relationship between the ACPC and front-line staff is variable, with many professionals seeing the ACPC as "... remote and out of touch" (Hallett, 1995, p 336) and many ACPC representatives undertaking little regular feedback of decisions to operational levels (Lupton et al, 1999b). Not least as a result of the difficulties of representation and accountability outlined above, the ACPC is seen by its members as having an only limited ability to effect operational change. While all involved expressed reservations about the capacity of the ACPC to influence the behaviour of its member organisations, it was NHS staff that were again seen, by both NHS and non-NHS ACPC members alike, to be least able to effect change at the local level. Views were mixed on the question of whether statutory status would enable the ACPC more effectively to determine the actions of its agency/professional members. Generally it was felt that, even with executive status, it would be difficult for the ACPC to override the organisational imperatives surrounding the operation of its constituent agencies. These imperatives (achieving key service objectives, ensuring public support and adequate funding and defending service paradigms) can be seen to represent the 'substructural' factors identified by Benson as influencing the superstructural dynamics of interorganisational networks such as the ACPC.

Equilibrium within provider networks

Domain consensus (who does what)

Despite the fairly detailed prescription of the *Working together* guidance on the roles of different players within the local provider networks, the evidence suggests that these networks are characterised by variable degrees of domain consensus. One of the generally perceived strengths of the ACPC is its ability to enhance mutual role understanding on the part of its disparate agency/professional members. Front-line workers also seem reasonably clear about the roles they perform and those performed by others. Some areas of confusion about NHS roles are, however, evident. Generally there is less certainty about the role of relatively infrequent health players within the network, such as accident and emergency doctors/nurses and paediatricians. There is also evidence of concerns about role demarcation, especially between the social worker and the heath visitor and the latter and the GP. In particular, there appears to be growing pressure on the fairly 'elastic' role of the health visitor to make a greater contribution to child protection, in addition to the increased demands of individual caseload and community development work. There is also some dissonance between the expectations held by a particular group about its role in child protection and the perception that fellow professionals have of that role. This is most clearly the case with GPs, who are accorded, both within government guidance and by fellow professionals, a much more pivotal role in all stages of the child protection process than they typically assume for themselves. With the exception of the role of the GP, however, the consensus about who does what in child protection appears to be relatively strong at both strategic and local levels.

Ideological consensus (how it is done)

This appears to be the biggest area of potential disequilibrium within the local provider networks. Tensions are evident at both ACPC and front-line levels as a result of the clash of different organisational and/or disciplinary 'paradigms'. Despite the attempt of central practice guidance to assert the multiagency ownership of the ACPC, for example, there remains a perception on the part of its NHS membership that it is dominated by the investigation-focused preoccupations of social services and the police (Sanders et al, 1997). Among NHS professionals, a distinction may be drawn between those, such as child psychiatric services or accident and emergency services, that are mainly focused on treatment or prevention, and those, such as general practice, paediatrics and, increasingly health visiting, that may also have a role to play in investigation. Those with broader child welfare or therapeutic concerns, such as education, mental health services and midwifery, may be less likely to view the operation of the ACPC as directly relevant to their organisational/ professional priorities.

This ideological dissonance is reflected at front-line level. Evidence suggests that there is considerable tension within the local network as a result of diverse disciplinary or organisational views of both of the nature of the client/problem and of the appropriate response. In particular, different service ideologies are characterised by variations in terms of thresholds for intervention and in the balance seen to obtain between prevention and protection. Such tensions may be played out within specific professional roles. Thus, health visitors may have difficulty in reconciling externally imposed expectations of family surveillance with more traditional disciplinary responsibilities for family support. Other professionals may experience deeper disciplinary, indeed epistemological, tensions. General practitioners, for example, may find it particularly difficult to balance a commitment to evidence-based knowledge with what they consider to be the more intuitive, experiential approaches of other front-line professionals (particularly social workers). Many health professionals, moreover, may have problems more generally with the diminished importance of the medical model occasioned by the policy shift from *child abuse* to that of *child protection*.

Positive evaluation (how well it is seen to be done by others)

There is evidence that the operation of ACPCs may be reasonably effective in encouraging a greater mutual positive evaluation on the part of their member agencies. This not only involves increased understanding of the practical and financial constraints under which other agencies operate, but also a more general appreciation of their different service paradigms and priorities (substructural imperatives). Much, of course, depends on the particular agencies participating in the ACPC, the strength of their relationships as well as the individual personalities involved. However strong the level of mutual positive evaluation between strategic level staff, moreover, this may not be reflected at the front line. The uneven nature of the relationship between the ACPC and front-line staff, described earlier, may limit the extent to which these positive evaluations are transmitted to front-line professionals.

At operational level, there are indications that the extent of positive evaluation may be more mixed than at strategic level. In general, it is likely to be higher between NHS sub-groups than between non-health professionals and their health colleagues. Equilibrium on this dimension is clearly affected by the extent to which different professional groups actually work together, with negative stereotypical assumptions or prejudices about each other being more likely on the part of those who only infrequently collaborate (Blyth and Milner, 1990). Thus, the lower levels of positive evaluation generally expressed by non-NHS professionals in respect of the performance of accident and emergency doctors and hospital paediatricians, compared with that of health visitors and school nurses, can be related to the relative infrequency with which they encounter such staff. Low positive evaluations also stem from the disjunction between role expectation and role performance. The almost universally low evaluation of the role of GPs in child protection, for example, on the part of health and non-health colleagues alike, derives from the fact that GPs are not performing their role in the way that others, including the central policy community, anticipate.

Work coordination (the practical arrangements for doing it)

Differences in terms of the working practices of different agencies and professional groups may also serve to undermine the equilibrium of local provider networks. Discrepancies in the financial and planning cycles of participating agencies, in particular, are seen to affect the strategic decision-making capacity of the ACPC. Time pressures on members, particularly those belonging to more than one ACPC, also appear to inhibit effective participation. At the operational level, considerable tensions are evident as a result of workload and time management differences on the part of different professional groups. Thus the very different working environment of accident and emergency doctors and GPs, with a high turnover of patients and minimal consultation times, compared with those of social workers and, to an extent, health visitors, is seen to constrain their role in child protection. Frustration also results from different organisational practices around, for example, the communication of relevant information to professionals in other agencies. Again, while these difficulties are seen to affect many health professional groups, they are most commonly identified in respect of the GP. The participation of GPs within the child protection conference appears to be constrained by a range of practical considerations, including financial disincentives to attend CPCs, reduced 'ownership' of patient lists, fewer home visits, the use of locums for on-call services, and shorter consultation times.

In combination, therefore, the local child protection provider networks appear to be characterised by uneven performance on the four dimensions listed by Benson (1975). Not least as a result of the prescriptions of central guidance, provider networks display a reasonably good understanding and acceptance of each other's roles in child protection (*domain consensus*). This is particularly true at the strategic level and among those front-line professionals who work together most frequently. Partly due to the variable nature of the relationship between the ACPC and operational levels, however, and the obduracy of wider service and disciplinary paradigms, agreement is less apparent on the nature of child protection work (*ideological consensus*). Disagreement is evident at both strategic and front-line levels about the thresholds for intervention and the appropriate forms of treatment or response. The achievement of both domain and ideological consensus is not assisted by practical tensions in workload/time management and different organisational practices (*work coordination*). Despite the impact of government guidance, these factors combine to undermine the perceived value of different agency/professional contributions to the child protection network (*positive evaluation*). As with domain consensus, the condition of positive evaluation is stronger at strategic than at front-line level. This particular combination of attributes means that the child protection provider networks are difficult to fit exactly into Benson's key types of interorganisational equilibrium. An extension of his typology would suggest that they most closely approximate the condition of *domain inefficiency*: reasonably strong domain consensus, weaker ideological consensus, variable degrees of positive evaluation and poor work coordination.

Thoughts for the future

The historical analysis of attempted collaboration between health and social care services reveals an only limited degree of success. Commentators suggest that this is due to an emphasis on the mechanisms or procedures of collaboration rather than on creating the incentives for different agencies and professional groups to work together (Hudson, 1992). The problem with much central policy has been the assumption that agencies with very different organisational priorities and cultures are somehow naturally inclined to cooperate. This has ignored the impact of what Benson terms 'sub-structural' factors on the dynamics of collaboration. Our examination of the child protection system suggests that similar assumptions have been made and similar difficulties obtain. At both strategic and operational levels there is evidence that the effective operation of child protection networks is constrained by deeper 'imperatives' affecting agency/ professional behaviour. These imperatives derive from factors both internal and external to the network.

Internally, the implementation of the centrally driven 'coordination mandate' may be undermined by resistance to knowledge sharing or knowledge adjustment on the part of some front-line staff and by the differential social and, therefore, disciplinary, power and influence of the professional groups involved. Other potential tensions are introduced by different patterns of accountability and governance within participating organisations and by the different physical structures and cultures of the agencies involved. Further 'sub-structural' factors influencing the behaviour of network members derive from the pursuit of different core service objectives, from defensiveness around organisational paradigms, and from the need to secure sufficient resources and public legitimacy. Externally, the equilibrium of the provider network is affected by knowledge shifts or changing power balances within the policy sector, or society, more widely. Most critical has been the challenge to effective interprofessional collaboration presented by the almost continuous process of reorganisation of the public sector during the 1970s, 1980s and 1990s.

As an organisation, the NHS may experience particular problems within a multiagency/professional process such as child protection. These stem especially from the fragmented nature of the service and from the adverse impact on within-service, as well as external, collaboration of the (hitherto) competitive ethos of the internal market. Arguably, more than any other public sector agency, the NHS has suffered from historic internal divisions and rivalries between its constituent professional groups, and between central and local as well as professional and managerial lines of accountability. The relative power of its medical professionals has enabled them to resist attempts at centrally imposed practice frameworks and exhortations to more collaborative ways of working. In particular, the mechanisms of mandated coordination have had only limited impact on the activities of those groups, such as GPs, which have historically enjoyed considerable operational autonomy.

This book, however, has also identified signs of potentially positive change, at both central and local levels, that may serve to counter some of the negative tendencies identified by the foregoing analysis. At a central level, the attempt to replace the competitive ethos of the internal market with a more collaborative approach, reflected in the 1999 Health Act and the 2000 *NHS Plan* (DoH, 2000a) may, if successful, help to overcome some of the barriers to collaboration between purchasers and providers. Continued policy pressure towards more 'cross-cutting' approaches between the NHS and other agencies, particularly local authorities (*Modernising social services*, DoH, 1998a; *Modern local government*, DETR, 1998) is underpinned by the development of national service frameworks and 'joined-up' initiatives such as *Sure Start*, joint children's services plans, Connexions, and health improvement programmes. Collaboration is also enabled by the 'flexibilities' (pooled budgets, lead commissioning and integrated working) of the 1999 Health Act. Perhaps most importantly, given the need to provide the motivations rather than just the mechanisms (or exhortations) to collaborate, these enabling mechanisms are underpinned by the financial incentives of the Modernisation Fund and the children's services grant. The reform of the regulatory system, with the creation of the National Care Standards Commission and tighter performance management via the new performance assessment frameworks may also serve as levers for greater collaboration.

At a local level, these changes may lessen some of the tensions within the ACPC and front-line networks resulting from differences in work coordination and service priorities as well as from varying forms of governance and accountability. In particular, if they are sufficiently resourced, the development of the designated and named professional roles may assist in the representation of the NHS within local networks and enhance the degree of ideological consensus and positive evaluation across the service and between NHS and non-NHS professionals. Greater consistency of practice may also be enabled by the revised and extended 1999 version of the *Working together* guidance and by the implementation of the new *Framework for the assessment of children and their families* (DoH et al, 2000).

In respect of the role of the NHS more specifically, much may depend on the contribution made by the PCGs/PCTs to the ACPCs and local provider networks. As we write, the nature of this contribution remains uncertain. On the one hand, the introduction of the PCGs/PCTs may deliver a corporate capacity for GPs within multiagency forums such as the ACPC, and possibly introduce a greater degree of local democratic accountability to primary healthcare services. The strong professional influence of GPs may be mitigated somewhat by the performance frameworks surrounding the operation of the PCG/PCT boards, and by the presence of representatives of other groups/agencies. On the other hand, the generally strengthened hand of GPs vis-à-vis other professional sub-groups may simply reinforce already unequal relations of power within the 'micro politics' of local networks. Early evidence suggests that the influence of non-NHS representatives on the PCGs/PCTs may not be extensive (Glendinning and Coleman, 2000). Moreover, although the PCGs/PCTs are empowered to represent the interests of GPs as a whole, their decisions hold only limited sway over the actions of individual local practices. Finally, the more that GPs are absorbed into the governance of the NHS, the more their particular professional concerns and priorities will be reinforced within the service as a whole. On present evidence, the likelihood that this will result in higher prominence to child protection services does not appear to be strong.

This book has explicitly set out to examine the 'fault-lines' or tensions within the child protection system and to identify factors which, despite the best of intentions on the part of individual professionals and/or their agencies, serve to undermine both process and outcome in interprofessional, multiagency work. Against the rather pessimistic scenario outlined above, however, it must be acknowledged that, due to the quality of local procedures, good working relationships established over time and the commitment of individuals and their agencies, the bulk of local interagency/interprofessional work delivers good outcomes for children and their families.

Very occasionally, as with the tragedy of Anna Climbie, the system breaks down. This may be the result of role confusion, lack of work cooperation and/or limited ideological consensus on the part of the professionals and agencies involved. It will almost certainly, however, as with many such cases before it (Reder et al, 1993), raise questions about the adequacy of available resources, including training and staff support. In this respect the concluding paragraph of Hallett's research, undertaken nearly 10 years ago, remains as pertinent today:

> ... the child welfare needs of children and families need to be met through accessible, supportive, non-stigmatising and *available* services, which requires a commitment to providing the resources to ... promote welfare as well as to undertake routinised, defensive case management. (Hallett, 1995, p 347; original emphasis)

References

6, Perri (1997) *Holistic government*, London: Demos.

Abbott, A. (1995) 'Boundaries of social work or social work boundaries?', *Social Services Review*, vol 69, no 4, pp 545-62.

ADSS (Association of Directors of Social Services) (1999) *Good practice guidelines: Social services officer nominees on Primary Care Groups*, London: ADSS.

Agass, M., Coulter, A., Mant, J. and Fuller, A. (1991) 'Patient participation in general practice: who participates?', *British Journal of General Practice*, vol 41, pp 198-201.

Aldridge, M. (1999) 'Dragged to market: being a professional in the postmodern world', *British Journal of Social Work*, vol 26, pp 177-94.

Alford, R. (1975) *Health care politics*, Chicago, IL: University of Chicago.

Allsop, J. (1984) *Health policy and the National Health Service*, London: Longman.

Alvesson, M. (1993) 'Organisation as rhetoric: knowledge-intensive forms and the strugle with ambiguity', *Journal of Management Studies*, vol 30, no 6, pp 997-1015.

Armstrong, H. (1995) *Annual Reports of Child Protection Committees 1993/ 94*, Report No 1, London: ACPC Series.

Armstrong, H. (1996) *Annual Reports of Child Protection Committees 1994/ 95*, London: ACPC Series.

Atkinson, P. (1995) *Medical talk and medical work*, London: Sage Publications.

Audit Commission (1986a) *Developing community care for adults with mental handicap*, Occasional Paper 9, London: HMSO.

Audit Commission (1986b) *Making a reality of community care*, London: HMSO.

Audit Commission (1992) *Homeward bound: A new course for community health*, London: HMSO.

Audit Commission (1994) *Seen but not heard: Co-ordinating community child health and social services for children in need*, London: DoH.

Bachrach, P. and Baratz, M.S. (1970) *Power and poverty*, New York, NY: Oxford University Press.

Bair, J. (1997) *Foundations for enterprise knowledge management*, London: Garner Group Strategic Analysis Report.

Barker, R.W. (1996) 'Child protection, public services and the chimera of market force efficiency', *Children & Society*, vol 10, pp 28-39.

Barnett, R (1994) *The limits of competence: Knowledge, higher education and society*, Buckingham: Open University Press.

Barrett, S. and Fudge, C. (eds) (1981) *Policy and action*, London: Methuen.

Benson, J.K. (1975) 'The interorganisational network as a political economy', *Administrative Science Quarterly*, vol 20, pp 229-49.

Benson, J.K. (1983) 'A framework for policy analysis', in D.L. Rogers and D.A. Whetton (eds) *Interorganisational coordination*, Ames, IA: Iowa State University Press.

Bernstein, B. (1990) *Class, codes and control*, London: Sage Publications.

Birchall, E. (1992) *Report to the Department of Health: Working together in child protection: Report of Phase Two: A survey of the experience and perceptions of six key professions*, Stirling: University of Stirling.

Birchall, E. with Hallett, C. (1995) *Working together in child protection: Report of Phase Two: A survey of the experience and perceptions of six key professions*, London: HMSO.

Blackler, F. (1995) 'Knowledge, knowledge works and organisation: an overview and interpretation', *Organisation Studies*, vol 16, pp 1021-46.

Blumenthal, I. (1994) *Child abuse: A handbook for health practitioners*, London: Edward Arnold.

Blyth, E. and Milner, M.J. (1990) 'The process of interagency work' in The Violence Against Children Study Group, *Taking child abuse seriously*, London: Unwin Hyman.

Booth, T.A. (1981) 'Collaboration between the health and social services: Part 1, a case study of joint care planning', *Policy & Politics*, vol 9, no 1, pp 23-49.

Broussine, M., Cox, P. and Davies, F. (1988) 'The significance of interprofessional stereotyping in the health and social services', *Local Government Studies*, vol 14, no 3, pp 57-67.

Brown, I. (1997) 'A skill mix parent support initiative in health visiting: an evaluation study', *Health Visitor*, vol 70, no 9, pp 339-43.

Brown, R.G.S. (1975) *The management of welfare*, Glasgow: Fontana.

Buckley, H. (1999) 'Child protection practice: an ungovernable enterprise?', *Economic & Social Review*, vol 30, no 1, pp 21-40.

Burgner, T. (1996) *The regulation and inspection of social services*, London: The Stationery Office.

Burton, K. (1996) *Child protection issues in general practice*, Report commissioned by South Essex Health Authority, Essex Social Services Child Protection Committee, Essex: Essex County Council.

Butcher, T. (1995) *Delivering welfare: The governance of the social services in the 1990s*, Buckingham: Open University Press.

Butler, J.R. (1997) 'Child health surveillance in England and Wales: the good news', *Child: Care, Health and Development*, vol 23, no 4, pp 327-37.

Cabinet Office (1999) *Modernising government*, Cm 4310, London: The Stationery Office.

Caddick, J., Jermansen, K., Mastrottaro, J. and Senecah, S. (1999) 'Conflict assessment and the Cape Cod national seashore', *Mediation Quarterly*, vol 17, no 1, pp 21-40.

Carnell, J., Sackman, T., Botes, S. and Jackson, P. (1999) 'Leading the future', *Community Practitioner*, vol 72, no 9, pp 280-2.

Carrier, J. and Kendall, I. (1998) *Health and the National Health Service*, London: Athlone Press.

Cawson, A. (1986) *Corporation and political theory*, Oxford: Blackwell.

Challis, L., Fuller, S., Henwood, M., Klein, R., Plowden, W., Webb, A., Whittingham, P. and Wistow, G. (1988) *Joint approaches to social policy: Rationality and practice*, Cambridge: Cambridge University Press.

Chambers, R. and Belcher, J. (1993) 'Work patterns of general practitioners before and after the introduction of the 1990 contract', *British Journal of General Practice*, vol 43, pp 410-12.

Chan, P.A. and Rudman, M.J. (1998) 'Paradigms for mental health nursing: fragmentation or integration?', *Journal of Psychiatric and Mental Health Nursing*, vol 5, pp 143-6.

Chapman, T., Hugman, R. and Williams, A. (1995) 'Effectiveness of interprofessional relationships: a case illustration of joint working', in K. Soothill, L. Mackay and C. Webb (eds) *Interprofessional relations in health care*, London: Edward Arnold, pp 46-61.

Chisholm, J. (1998a) Chair of GMSC's letter to membership on the subject of Primary Care Groups, London: BMA.

Chisholm, J (1998b) 'Primary care and the NHS White Papers', *British Medical Journal*, vol 316, pp 1687-8.

Clarke, J., Cochrane, A. and McLaughlin, E. (eds) (1994) *Managing social policy*, Buckingham: Open University Press.

Clay, T. (1989) 'Nursing and politics: the unquiet relationship', in M. Jolley and P. Allen (eds) *Current issues in nursing*, London: Chapman and Hall.

Clyde, Lord (1992) *The Report of the Inquiry into the Removal of Children from Orkney in February 1991* (The Clyde Report), Edinburgh: HMSO.

Collins, H.M. (1990) *Artificial experts: Social knowledge and intelligent machines*, Cambridge, MA/London: MIT Press.

Coote, A. and Hunter, D.J. (1996) *A new agenda for health*, London: Institute for Public Policy Research.

Cope, S. and Goodship, J. (1999) 'Regulating collaborative government: towards joined-up government', *Public Policy and Administration*, vol 14, no 2, pp 3-15.

Court Committee (1976) *Fit for the future: Report of the Court Committee on Child Health Services*, London: HMSO.

Craig, P.M. and Smith, L.N. (1998) 'Health visiting and public health: back to our roots or a new branch?', *Health and Social Care in the Community*, vol 6, no 3, pp 172-80.

Crane, A. (1998) 'Culture clash and mediation: exploring the cultural dynamics of business–NGO collaboration', *Greener Management International Journal*, vol 24, no 5, pp 61-76.

Currey, L. and Werquin, J. and Associates (1993) *Educating professionals: Responding to new expectations for competence and accountability*, San Fransico, CA: Jossey Bass.

Cunningham, C. (1992) 'Sea defences: a professional network?', in D. Marsh and R.A.W. Rhodes (eds) *Policy networks in British government*, Oxford: Clarendon Press.

Cutler, T. and Waine, B. (1994) *Managing the welfare state*, Oxford: Berg.

Dalley, G. (1991) 'Beliefs and behaviour: professionals and the policy process', *Journal of Ageing Studies*, vol 5, no 2, pp 163-80.

Daugbjerg, C. and Marsh, D. (1998) 'Explaining policy outcomes: integrating the policy network approach with macro-level and micro-level analysis', in D. Marsh (ed) *Comparing policy networks*, Buckingham: Open University Press.

Davenport, T. and Prusack, L. (1998) *Working knowledge: How organisations manage what they know best*, Boston, MA: Harvard Business School Press.

Day, P. and Klein, R. (1987) *Accountabilities: Five public services*, London: Tavistock.

Day, P. and Klein, R. (1997) *Steering but not rowing: The transformation of the Department of Health*, Bristol: The Policy Press.

DETR (Department of the Environment, Transport and the Regions) (1998) *Modern local government: In touch with the people*, Cm 4014, London: The Stationery Office.

DHSS (Department of Health and Social Security) (1971) *Better services for the mentally handicapped*, Cmnd 4683, London: HMSO.

DHSS (1974) *Report of the Committee of Inquiry into the care and supervision provided in relation to Maria Colwell*, London: HMSO.

DHSS (1975) *Better services for the mentally ill*, Cmnd 6223, London: HMSO.

DHSS (1976) *Non-accidental injury to children*, Area Review Committees, LASSL (76) 2.

DHSS (1980) *Child abuse: Central register systems*, LASSL (80) 4.

DHSS (1982) *Child abuse: A study of inquiry reports 1973-1981*, London: HMSO.

DHSS (1983) *NHS management inquiry* (Griffiths Report), London: HMSO.

DHSS (1988a) *Diagnosis of child sexual abuse: Guidance for doctors*, London: HMSO.

DHSS (1988b) *Child protection: Guidance for senior nurses, health visitors and midwives*, London HMSO.

DHSS and Welsh Office (1988) *Working together: A guide to arrangements for inter-agency co-operation for the protection of children from abuse*, London: HMSO.

Dobson, J. (1992) 'Wall demands Department of Health guidance on cash for community care', *Health Service Journal*, 8 October, p 7.

DoH (Department of Health) (1989a) *Working for patients*, Cm 555, London: HMSO.

DoH (1989b) *Caring for people: Community care in the next decade and beyond*, Cm 849, London: HMSO.

DoH (1990) *Community care in the next decade and beyond: Policy guidance*, London: HMSO.

DoH (1991) *Child abuse: A study of inquiring reports 1980-1989*, London: HMSO.

DoH (1992a) *Children's service plans*, LAC(92) 18, London: HMSO.

DoH (1992b) *Child protection: Guidance for senior nurses, health visitors and midwives*, London: HMSO.

DoH (1992c) *The health of the nation*, London: HMSO.

DoH (1995a) *Child protection: Messages from research*, London: HMSO.

DoH (1995b) *Child protection: Clarification of arrangements between the NHS and other agencies*, London: HMSO.

DoH (1996) *Child protection: Medical responsibilities: Guidance to doctors working with child protection agencies: Addendum to Working together under the Children Act 1989*, London: HMSO.

DoH (1997) *The new NHS: Modern, dependable*, Cm 3807, London: The Stationery Office.

DoH (1998a) *Modernising social services: Promoting independence, improving protection, raising standards*, Cm 4169, London: The Stationery Office.

DoH (1998b) *Working together to safeguard children: New government proposals for inter-agency co-operation*, Consultation Paper, London: Children's Services Branch, DoH.

DoH (1998c) *Quality Protects: Framework for action*, London: DoH Social Care Group.

DoH (1999a) 'Government issues guidance on protecting children', Press release, no 0514.

DoH (1999b) *Saving lives: Our healthier nation*, Cm 4386, London: The Stationery Office.

DoH, DfEE and Home Office (2000) *Framework for the assessment of children in need and their families*, London: The Stationery Office.

DoH (2000a) *The NHS Plan: A plan for investement, a plan for reform*, Cm 4818-1, London: The Stationery Office.

DoH (2000b) *Making a difference*, London: The Stationery Office.

DoH and SSI (Social Services Inspectorate) (1990a) *Inspection of child protection services in Rochdale*, Manchester: DoII/SSI, NW Region.

DoH and SSI (1990b) *Report of an inspection of collaborative working arrangements between child protection agencies in Cleveland*, London: HMSO.

DoH and SSI (1995) *The challenge of partnership in child protection: Practice guide*, London: HMSO.

DoH and SSI (1996) *Working with child sexual abuse. Department of Health guidelines for trainers and managers in social services departments*, London: HMSO.

DoH and Standing Nursing and Midwifery Advisory Committee (1997) *Child protection: Guidance for senior nurses, health visitors and their managers*, London: The Stationery Office.

DoH and Welsh Office (1995) *Child protection: Clarification of arrangements between the NHS and other agencies: Addendum to Working together under the Children Act 1989*, London: HMSO.

DoH and Welsh Office (1998) *Putting patients first*, London: The Stationery Office.

DoH, Home Office, DfEE (Department for Education and Employment) (1999) *Working together to safeguard children: A guide to inter-agency working to safeguard and promote the welfare of children*, London: The Stationery Office.

Doig, A. (1995) 'Mixed signals? Public sector change and the proper conduct of public business', *Public Administration*, vol 73, pp 191-212.

Dominelli, L. (1996) 'Deprofessionalising social work: anti-oppressive practice, competencies, postmodern', *British Journal of Social Work*, vol 26, pp 153-75.

Donaldson, L.J. and Cresswell, P.A. (1994) 'The NHS reforms and child protection', *Health and Social Care in the Community*, vol 2, no 4, pp 255-7.

Dowding, K. (1994) 'Policy networks: don't stretch a good idea too far', in P. Dunleavy and J. Stanyer (eds) *Contemporary political studies*, Belfast: Political Studies Association.

Dowding, K. (1995) 'Model or metaphor? A critical review of the policy network approach', *Political Studies*, vol 43, no 2, pp 136-58.

Dunnell, K. and Dobbs, J. (1982) *Nurses working in the community*, London: HMSO.

Duke, S., Macey, P. and Kiras, N. (1999) *Knowledge management*, Report Series vol 1, Hull: Butler Consulting Group.

Eckstein, H. (1958) *The English health service*, Cambridge, MA: Harvard University Press.

Etzioni, A. (ed) (1969) *The semi-professions and their organisations: Teachers, nurses and social workers*, New York, NY: The Free Press.

Fairclough, N. (1989) *Language of power*, London: Longman.

Farmer, E. and Owen, M. (1995) *Child protection practice: Private risks and public remedies. A study of decision-making, intervention and outcome in child protection work*, London: HMSO.

Fletcher, G.J.O. and Fitness, J. (1996) *Knowledge structures in close relationships: A social psychological approach*, New Jersey, NJ: Lawrence Erlbaum Associates.

Fox, S. and Dingwall, R. (1985) 'An exploratory study of variations in social workers' and health visitors' definition of child mistreatment', *British Journal of Social Work*, vol 15, no 5, pp 467-78.

Friedson, E. (1970) *Profession of medicine: A study of the sociology of applied knowledge*, New York, NY: Mead & Co, Dodd.

Gabe, J., Kelleher, D. and Williams, G. (eds) (1994) *Challenging medicine*, London: Routledge.

Gibbons, J., Conroy, S. and Bell, C. (1995) *Operating the child protection system: A study of child protection practices in English local authorities. Studies in child protection*, London: HMSO.

Giddens, A. (1991) *Modernity and self-identity: Self and society in the late modern age*, Cambridge: Polity.

Glendinning, C. and Coleman, A. (2000) 'Taking your partners: developing relationships between primary care groups and local authorities', *Research Policy & Planning*, vol 18, no 3, pp 25-33.

Glennerster, H., Korman, N. and Marsden-Wilson, F. (1983) *Planning for priority groups*, London: Blackwell.

GMSC (General Medical Services Committee) (1996) *Core services: Taking the initiative*, London: BMA.

Goffman, E. (1974) *Frame analysis: An essay on the organisation of experience*, New York, NY: Harper and Row.

Goodwin, S. (1994) 'Purchasing effective care for parents and young children', *Health Visitor*, vol 67, no 4, pp 127-9.

Gough, I. (1979) *The political economy of the welfare state*, London: Macmillan.

Griffiths, R. (1988) *Community care: Agenda for action*, London: HMSO.

Gusfield, J.R. (1989) 'Constructing the ownership of social problems: fun and profit in the welfare state', *Social Problems*, vol 36, no 5, pp 416-30.

Guy, P. (1994) 'A General Social Work Council – a critical look at the issues', *British Journal of Social Work*, vol 24, pp 261-71.

Hallett, C. (1995) *Interagency co-ordination in child protection: Studies in child protection*, London: HMSO.

Hallett, C. and Birchall, E. (1992) *Co-ordination and child protection: A review of the literature*, Edinburgh: HMSO.

Hallett, C. and Stevenson, O. (1980) *Child abuse: Aspects of interprofessional co-operation*, London: HMSO.

Ham, C. (1981) *Policy making in the NHS*, London: Macmillan.

Ham, C. (1999) *Health policy in Britain* (4th edn), Basingstoke: Macmillan.

Ham, C. and Hill, M. (1984) *The policy process in the modern capitalist state*, Brighton: Wheatsheaf.

Hannay, D., Usherwood, T. and Platts, M. (1992) 'Workload of general practitioners before and after the new contract', *British Medical Journal*, vol 304, pp 615-18.

Harrison, S. and Pollitt, C. (1994) *Controlling health professionals*, Buckingham: Open University Press.

Harrison, S., Hunter, D.J., Marnoch, G. and Pollitt, C. (1989) 'General management and medical autonomy in the National Health Service', *Health Services Management Research*, vol 2, no 1, pp 38-46.

Hausman, D. and Le Grand, J. (1999) 'Incentives and health policy: primary and secondary care in the British National Health Service', *Social Science and Medicine*, vol 49, pp 1299-307.

Hay, C. (1998) 'The tangled webs we weave: the discourse, strategy and practice of networking', in D. Marsh (ed) *Comparing policy networks*, Buckingham: Open University Press.

Haywood, S. and Alaszewski, A. (1980) *Crisis in the health service*, London: Croom Helm.

Haywood, S. and Hunter, D. (1982) 'Consultative processes in health policy in the United Kingdom: a view from the centre', *Public Administration*, vol 69, pp 143-62.

Heclo, H. (1978) 'Issue networks in the executive establishment', in A. King (ed) *The new American political system*, Washington, DC: American Enterprise Institute.

Hehir, B. (1998) 'Big mother is watching you', *Nursing Times*, vol 94, no 41, pp 38-9.

Hiscock, J. and Pearson, M. (1995) *Perspectives on the impact of GP fundholding on community care and child protection*, Liverpool: Health and Community Care Research Unit, University of Liverpool.

Hoggett, P. (1991) 'A new management in the public sector?', *Policy & Politics*, vol 19, no 4, pp 243-6.

Home Office (1950) *Joint circular with Ministry of Health and Ministry of Education: Children neglected or ill-treated in their own homes*, London: HMSO.

Home Office (1996) *On the record: The government's proposals for access to criminal records for employment and related purposes in England and Wales*, London: HMSO.

Home Office and DoH (1992) *Memorandum of good practice on video recorded interviews with child witnesses for criminal proceedings*, London: HMSO.

Home Office, DoH, DES (Department of Education and Science) and Welsh Office (1991) *Working together under the Children Act, 1989*, London: HMSO.

Honigsbaum, F. (1989) *Health, happiness and security: The creation of the National Health Service*, London: Routledge.

Hood, C. (1995) 'Contemporary public management: a new global paradigm?', *Public Policy and Administration*, vol 10, no 2, pp 104-17.

Howe, D. (1992) 'Child abuse and the bureaucratisation of social work', *The Sociological Review*, vol 38, pp 491-508.

Hoyte, P. (1996) 'Protecting the paediatrician: responding to recrimination', *Child Abuse Review*, vol 5, no 2, pp 103-12.

Hudson, B. (1992) 'Quasi-markets in health and social care in Britain: can the public sector respond?', *Policy & Politics*, vol 20, no 2, pp 131-42.

Hudson, B. (1994) 'General practice and community care: developing the links', *Health and Social Care in the Community*, vol 2, no 5, pp 309-21.

Hudson, B. (1997) 'Caring sharing', *Community Care*, September/October, pp 2-3.

Hudson, B. (1998) 'Circumstances change cases: local government and the NHS', *Social Policy and Administration*, vol 32, no 1, pp 71-86.

Hudson, B. (2000) 'Social services and primary care groups: a window of collaborative opportunity?', *Health and Social Care in the Community*, vol 8, no 4, pp 242-50.

Hughes, G., Mears, R. and Winch, C. (1997) 'An inspector calls? Regulation and accountability in the public services', *Policy & Politics*, vol 25, no 3, pp 299-313.

Hugman, R. (1991) 'Organization and professionalism: the social work agenda in the 1990s', *British Journal of Social Work*, vol 21, pp 199-216.

Hunter, D. (1980) *Coping with uncertainty*, Chichester: Research Studies Press.

Hunter, D. (1994) 'From tribalism to corporatism: the managerial challenge to medical dominance', in J. Gabe, D. Kelleher and G. Williams (eds) *Challenging medicine*, London: Routledge.

Hunter, D. and Wistow, G. (1987) 'Community care in Britain', *Sociology of Health and Illness*, vol 10, no 3, pp 311-13.

Ichijo, K., von Krogh, G. and Nonako, I. (1998) 'Knowledge enablers', in G. von Krogh, J. Roos and D. Kleine (eds) *Knowing in firms: Understanding, managing and measuring knowledge*, London: Sage Publications.

Ives, W., Gifford, T. and Hankins, D. (1998) 'Integrating knowledge and skills management', *ACM Groupware Bulletin*, vol 19, no 1, pp 51-3.

Jackson, S., Sanders, R. and Thomas, N. (1994) *Protecting children in Wales: The role and effectiveness of Area Child Protection Committees*, Swansea: University of Wales, Swansea.

Jamous, H. and Peloille, B. (1970) 'Changes in a French university–hospital system', in J. Jackson (ed) *Professions and professionalization*, Cambridge: Cambridge University Press.

Johnson, T. (1972) *Professions and power*, London: Macmillan.

Jordan, A.G. (1981) 'Iron triangles, woolly corporatism and elastice nets: images of the policy process', *Journal of Public Policy*, vol 1, pp 95-123.

Jordan, A.G., Maloney, W. and McLaughlin, A. (1994) 'Characterising agricultural policy networks', *Public Administration*, vol 72, no 4, pp 505-26.

Kempe, S.J. and Kempe, C.H. (1978) *Child abuse*, London: Open Books.

Kendrick, K. (1995) 'Nurses and doctors: a problem of partnership', in K. Soothill, L. Mackay and C. Webb (eds) *Interprofessional relations in health care*, London: Edward Arnold.

Khan, P., Lupton, C. and North, N. (1999a) 'Doctors on board', *Health Management*, vol 2(a), pp 20-2.

Khan, P., Lupton, C., Lacey, D. and North, N. (1999b) 'Primary care groups and partnerships with social services departments', *Social Services Research*, no 3, pp 19-29.

Kikert, W.J.M., Klijn, E.H. and Koppenjan, J.F.M. (1997) 'Introduction: a management perspective on policy networks', in W.J.M. Kikert, E.H. Klijn and J.F.M. Koppenjan (eds) *Managing complex networks: Strategies for the public sector*, London: Sage Publications.

Klein, J.T. (1996) *Crossing boundaries: Knowledge, disciplinarity and interdisciplinarities*, Charlottesville, VA: University of Virginia Press.

Klein, R. (1989) *The politics of the National Health Service*, London: Longman.

Klein, R. (1995) *The new politics of the National Health Service* (3rd edn), London: Longman.

Klijn, E.H. (1997) 'Policy networks: an overview', in W.J. Kikert, E.H. Klijn and J.F.M. Koppenjan (eds) *Managing complex networks: Strategies for the public sector*, London: Sage Publications.

Lave, J. and Wenger, E. (1991) *Situated learning: Legitimate peripheral participation*, Cambridge: Cambridge University Press.

Leach, P. (1997) 'What price home visiting and family support?', *Health Visitor*, vol 70, no 2, pp 72-4.

Lea-Cox, C. and Hall, A. (1991) 'Attendance of general practitioners at child protection case conferences', *British Medical Journal*, vol 302, pp 1378-9.

Leathard, A. (1990) *Health care provision: Past, present and future*, London: Chapman and Hall.

Leathard, A. (1994) *Going interprofessional: Working together for health and welfare*, London: Routledge.

Leedham, I. and Wistow, G. (1992) *Community care and general practitioners*, Working Paper No 6, Leeds: Nuffield Institute.

Levy, A. and Kahan, B. (1991) *The Pindown experience and the protection of children*, Stafford: Staffordshire County Council.

Lewis, J. (1993) 'Community care: policy imperatives, joint planning and enabling authorities', *Journal of Interprofessional Care*, vol 7, no 1, pp 7-14.

Light, D. (1998) 'Managed care in a new key: Britain's strategies for the 1990s', *International Journal of Health Services*, vol 28, pp 427-44.

Lipsky, M. (1980) *Street level bureaucracy: Dilemmas of the individual public services*, New York, NY: Russell Sage.

Llewellyn, S. (1998) 'Boundary work: costing and caring in the social services', *Accounting, Organizations and Society*, vol 23, no 1, pp 23-47.

London Borough of Bexley (1982) *Report of the Panel of Inquiry into the death of Lucie Gates*, London: Borough of Bexley and Bexley Health Authority.

London Borough of Brent (1985) *A child in trust: The report of the Panel of Inquiry into the circumstances surrounding the death of Jasmine Beckford*, London: London Borough of Brent.

London Borough of Greenwich (1987) *A child in mind: The protection of children in a responsible society*, London: London Borough of Greenwich.

Lupton, C. and Khan, P. (1998) 'The role of health professionals in the child protection process', *Journal of Interprofessional Care*, vol 10, no 2, pp 209-23.

Lupton, C., Buckland, S. and Moon, G. (1995) 'Consumer involvement in health care purchasing: the role and influence of the community health councils', *Health and Social Care in the Community*, vol 3, no 4, pp 215-26.

Lupton, C., Khan, P. and North, N. (1999a) 'Kings of the hill?: collaboration between general practice and social services departments in the new NHS', *Community Care*, 25-31 March.

Lupton, C., Khan, P. and North, N. (2000) 'The role of the general practitioner in child protection', *British Journal of General Practice*, vol 50, pp 977-81.

Lupton, C., Peckham, S. and Taylor, P. (1998) *Managing public involvement in healthcare purchasing*, Buckingham: Open University Press.

Lupton, C., Khan, P., North, N. and Lacey, D (1999b) *The role of health professionals in the child protection process*, Portsmouth: Social Services Research and Information Unit, Report No 41, University of Portsmouth.

McDonald, A.L., Langford, I.H. and Bolero, N. (1997) 'The future of community nursing in the United Kingdom', *Journal of Advanced Nursing*, vol 26, pp 257-65.

Macdonald, G. and Roberts, H. (1995) *What works in early years? Effective intervention for children and their families in health, social welfare, education and child protection*, Ilford: Barnardo's.

Mackay, L. and Webb, C. (1993) (eds) *Interprofessional relations in health care*, London: Edward Arnold.

Marks, L. and Hunter, D. (1998) *The development of primary care groups: Policy into practice*, Birmingham: NHS Confederation.

Marr, A. (1995) *Ruling Britannia*, London: Penguin.

Marsh, D. (1992) 'Youth employment policy 1970-1990: towards the exclusion of the Trade Unions', in D. Marsh and R.A.W. Rhodes (eds) *Policy networks in British government*, Oxford: Clarendon Press.

Marsh, D. (ed) (1998) *Comparing policy networks*, Buckingham: Open University Press.

Marsh, D. and Rhodes, R.A.W. (1992) *Policy networks in British government*, Oxford: Clarendon Press.

Massey, A. (1993) *Managing the public sector. A comparative analysis of the United Kingdom and the United States*, Aldershot: Edward Elgar.

May, T. and Buck, M. (1998) 'Power, professionalism and organisational transformation', *Sociological Research Online*, vol 3, no 2 (www.socresonline.org.uk/socresonlin/3/2/5).

Mayntz, R. (1994) 'Modernisation and the logic of interorganisational networks', MIGPF Working Paper No 4, Cologne: Max Planck Institut für Gesellschaftsforschung.

Mill, J.S. (1993) *Utilitarianism, on liberty, considerations on representative government, remarks on Bentham's philosophy*, London: Everyman.

Ministry of Health (1962) *A hospital plan for England and Wales*, Cmnd 1604, London: HMSO.

Ministry of Health (1963) *Health and welfare: The development of community care*, Cmnd 1973, London: HMSO.

Ministry of Health (1966) *Report of the Committee on senior nursing staff structures* (Salmon Report), London: HMSO.

Moon, G. and Lupton, C. (1995) 'Within acceptable limits: health care provider perspectives on community health councils in the reformed British National Health Service', *Policy & Politics*, vol 23, no 4, pp 335-46.

Moon, G. and North, N. (2000) *Policy and place: General medical practice in the UK*, London: Macmillan.

Moore, W. (1992) 'May the force be with you', *Health Service Journal*, vol 9, November, pp 24-7.

Moran-Ellis, J., Stone, M. and Wilkins, R. (1993) *Health professionals and child protection: Risk assessment and referral in physical abuse and neglect*, Guildford: University of Surrey.

Morrison, T. (1997) 'Emotionally competent child protection organisations: fallacy, fiction or necessity?', in J. Bates, R. Pugh and N. Thompson (eds) *Protecting children: Challenges and change*, Aldershot: Arena.

Mostyn (Lord Williams of) (1996) *Childhood matters: Report of the National Commission of Inquiry into the Prevention of Child Abuse. Volume 1: The Report*, London: The Stationery Office.

Mulford, C. and Rogers, D. (1982) 'Definitions and models' in D. Rogers and D. Whetton (eds) *Interorganisational co-ordination: Theory, research and implementation*, Ames, IA: Iowa State University Press

Myles, S., Wyke, S., Popay, J., Scott, J., Campbell, A. and Girling, J. (1998) *Total purchasing and community and continuing care: Lessons for future policy developments in the NHS*, London: King's Fund.

Nairne, P. (1984) 'Parliamentary control and accountability', in R. Maxwell and N. Weaver (eds) *Patient participation in health*, London: King Edward's Hospital Fund for London.

National Audit Office (1987) *Community care developments: Report to the Comptroller and Auditor General*, HC108, London: HMSO.

Newman, J. and Clarke, J. (1994) 'Going about our business? The managerialism of public services', in J. Clarke, A. Cochrane and E. McLaughlin (eds) *Managing social policy*, London: Sage Publications.

NHS Executive (1998) *The new NHS: Modern, dependable: Developing primary care groups*, HSC 1998/139, Leeds: NHS Executive.

NHSME (NHS Management Executive) (1992) *Local voices: The views of local people in purchasing for health*, London: NHSME.

North, N., Lupton, C. and Khan, P. (1999) 'The new NHS: doctors and nurses in the driving seat?', *Nursing Times*, vol 94, no 33, pp 8-10.

North, N., Lupton, C. and Khan, P. (2000) 'Going with the grain? GPs and the new NHS', *Health and Social Care in the Community*, vol 7, no 6, pp 409-17.

Offe, C. (1975) 'The theory of the capitalist state and the problem of policy formation', in L. Lindberg, R. Alford, C. Crouch and C. Offe (eds) *Stress and contradiction in modern capitalism*, Lexiton, MA: Lexiton Books.

Office of Health Economics (2000) *Compendium of health statistics* (12th edn), London: Office of Health Economics.

Orkney Inquiry (1991) *Report of the Inquiry into the Removal of Children from Orkney in February 1991*, London: HMSO.

Osborne, D. and Gaebler, T. (1992) *Reinventing government*, Reading: Addison-Wesley.

Øvreteit, J., Mathias, P. and Thompson, T. (1997) *Interprofessional working for health and social care*, London: Macmillan.

Ouchi, W. (1980) 'Markets, bureaucracies and clans', *Administrative Science Quarterly*, vol 25, pp 129-41.

Ottewill, R. and Wall, A. (1990) *The growth and development of the community health services*, Sunderland: Business Education Publishers.

Owens, P. and Glennerster, H. (1990) *Nursing in conflict*, London: Macmillan.

Parry, N. and Parry, J. (1979) 'Social work, professionalism and the state', in N. Parr, M. Rustin and C. Satyamurti (eds) *Social work, professionalism and the state*, London: Edward Arnold.

Parton, N. (1985) *The politics of child abuse*, London: Macmillan.

Parton, N. (1991) *Governing the family: Child care, child protection and the state*, London: Macmillan.

Parton, N. (1994) 'Government, (post)modernity and social work', *British Journal of Social Work*, vol 24, pp 9-32.

Parton, N. and Otway, O. (1995) 'The contemporary state of child protection policy and practice in England and Wales', *Children and Youth Studies Review*, vol 17, nos 5/6, pp 559-617.

Parton, N., Thorpe, D. and Wattam, C. (1997) *Child protection: Risk and the moral order*, London: Macmillan.

Paton, C. (1992) 'Devolution and centralism in the National Health Service', *Social Policy and Administration*, vol 27, no 2, pp 83-108.

Peters, G. (1986) *American public policy*, Basingstoke: Macmillan.

Pollitt, C. (1990) *Managerialism and the public services: The Anglo-American experience*, Oxford: Blackwell.

Powell, M. (1999) 'New Labour and the third way in the British National Health Service', *International Journal of Health Services*, vol 29, no 2, pp 353-70.

RCGP (Royal College of General Practitioners) (2000) *Evidence from the Royal College of General Practitioners to the Health Committee Inquiry into Children's Health* (www.rcgp.org.uk/news/statemen/RCT002.asp).

Read, M. (1992) 'Policy networks and issue networks: the politics of smoking', in D. Marsh and R.A.W. Rhodes (eds) *Policy networks in British government*, Oxford: Clarendon Press.

Reder, P., Duncan, S. and Gray, M. (1993) *Beyond blame: Child abuse tragedies revisited*, London: Routledge.

Reich, R. (1991) *The work of nations: Preparing ourselves for 21st century capitalism*, London: Simon and Schuster.

Rhodes, R.A.W. (1981) *Control and power in central–local relations*, Aldershot: Gower.

Rhodes, R.A.W. (1988) *Beyond Westminster and Whitehall*, London: Unwin Hyman.

Rhodes, R.A.W. (1995) *The new governance: Governing without government*, Swindon: ESRC.

Rhodes, R.A.W. (1997) *Understanding governance*, Buckingham: Open University Press.

Richardson, J. and Jordan, G. (1979) *Governing under pressure*, Oxford: Martin Robinson.

Richey, C.A. and Roffman, R.A. (1999) 'On the sidelines of guidelines: future thoughts on the fit between clinical guidelines and social work practice', *Research on Social Work Practice*, vol 9, no 3, pp 311-21.

Rickford, F. (2000) 'Who is flying this plane?', *Community Care*, 10-25 October, issue no 1344, pp 20-1.

Robinson, R. and Hayter, P. (1992) *Why GPs choose not to apply as fundholders*, Southampton: IHPS, University of Southampton.

Royal Commission on the NHS (1979) *Report* (Merrison Committee), Cmnd 7615, London: HMSO.

Sadlar, C. (1994) 'Is working together falling apart?', *Health Visitor*, vol 67, no 8, pp 259-60.

Salter, B. (1998) *The politics of change in the health service*, Basingstoke: Macmillan.

Salter, B. and Salter, C. (1993) 'Theatre of the absurd', *Health Service Journal*, 11 November, pp 30-1.

Salvage, J. (1988) 'Professionalization – or struggle for survival? A consideration of current proposals for the reform of nursing in the United Kingdom', *Journal of Advanced Nursing*, vol 13, pp 515-19.

Sanders, R. (1999) *The management of child protection services: Context and change*, Aldershot: Ashgate Arena.

Sanders, R., Jackson, S. and Thomas, N. (1997) 'Degrees of involvement: the interaction of focus and commitment in Area Child Protection Committees', *British Journal of Social Work*, vol 27, pp 871-92.

Sarangi, S. (1998) 'Interprofessional case construction in social work: the evidential status of information and its reportability', *Text*, vol 18, no 2, pp 241-70.

Saward, M. (1997) 'In search of the hollow crown', in P. Weller, H. Bakvis and R.A.W. Rhodes (eds) *The hollow crown*, London: Macmillan.

Schmitter, P. (1979) 'Still the century of corboralism?', in P. Schmitter and G. Lehmbruch (eds) *Trends towards corporatist intermediation*, London: Sage Publications.

Schmitz, H. (2000) 'Does local co-operation matter? Evidence from industrial clusters in South Asia and Latin America', *Oxford Development Studies*, vol 28, no 3, pp 323-36.

Schon, D.A. (1983) *The reflective practitioner: How professionals think in action*, London: Temple Smithe.

Schutz, A. and Luckmann, T. (1973) *The structures of the life-world*, Evanston, IL: Northwestern University Press.

Scott, A. and Wordsworth, S. (1998) 'The effects of shifts in the balance of care on general practice workload', *Family Practice*, vol 16, no 1, pp 12-17.

Scottish Office DoH (1997) *Designed to care: Renewing the National Health Service in Scotland*, Cm 3811, Edinburgh: DoH.

Secretary of State for Health (1999) *The government's response to the Second Report of the Health Committee on Primary Care Groups*, Cm 4468, London: The Stationery Office.

Secretary of State for Social Services (1988) *Report of the Inquiry into child abuse in Cleveland*, Cm 412, London: HMSO.

Seebohm, F. (1968) *Report of the Committee on Local Authority and Allied Personal Social Services*, London: HMSO.

Select Committee of the House of Commons (1993) *Community care services*, London: HMSO.

Sheldon, B. (1998) 'Evidence-based social services: prospects and problems', *Research, Policy and Planning*, vol 16, no 2, pp 16-18.

Sheppard, M. (1995) 'Social work, social science and practice wisdom', *British Journal of Social Work*, vol 25, no 3, pp 265-94.

Simpson, C.H., Simpson, R.J., Power, K.G., Salter, A. and Williams, G.-J. (1994) 'GPs' and health visitors' participation in child protection case conferences', *Child Abuse Review*, vol 3, pp 211-30.

Smith, J. (2000) 'Primary care groups and trusts: stages in a process of organisational evolution', *Health Services Management Research*, vol 13, no 4, pp 223-30.

Smith, M.J. (1993) *Pressure, power and policy. Power networks and state autonomy in Britain and the United States*, London: Harvester Wheatsheaf.

Smith, S. (1998) 'Child protection: are we going backwards?', *Community Practitioner*, vol 71, no 3, pp 98-9.

Soothill, K., Mackay, L. and Webb, C. (1995) *Interprofessional relations in health care*, London: Edward Arnold.

SSI (Social Services Inspectorate) (1995) *Evaluating child protection services: Child inspections 1993/4 - overview report*, London: SSI.

SSI Wales (1996) *Area Child Protection Committees and local government reorganisation*, Cardiff: SSI Wales.

Stacey, M. (1988) *The sociology of health and healing*, London: Routledge.

Stevenson, O. (1989) 'Multi-disciplinary work in child protection', in O. Stevenson (ed) *Child abuse: Public policy and professional practice*, London: Harvester Wheatsheaf.

Stewart, J. (1992) 'The rebuilding of public accountability', in J. Stewart, N. Lewis and D. Longley, *Accountability to the public*, London: European Policy Forum.

Stewart, J. (1995) *Innovation in democratic practice*, Birmingham: Institute of Local Government Studies, Birmingham University.

Stewart, J. and Walsh, K. (1992) 'Change in the management of public services', *Public Administration*, vol 70, pp 499-518.

Stoker, G. (1991) *The politics of local government*, Basingstoke: Macmillan.

Strauss, A., Schatzman, L., Ehrlich, D., Bucher, R. and Sabshin, M. (1963) 'The hospital and its negotiated order', in E. Friedson, *The hospital in modern society*, Basingstoke: Macmillan.

Strong, P. and Robinson, J. (1990) *The NHS under new management*, Buckingham: Open University Press.

Suchman, L.A. (1987) *Plans and situated actions: The problem of human machine communication*, Cambridge: Cambridge University Press.

Sutton, P. (1995) *Crossing the boundaries: A discussion of Children's Services Plans*, London: National Children's Bureau.

Symonds, A. (1997) 'Ties that bind: problems with GP-attachment', *Health Visitor*, vol 70, no 2, pp 53-5.

Taylor, S. and Tilley, N. (1989) 'Health visitors and child protection: conflict, contradictions and ethical dilemmas', *Health Visitor*, vol 62, no 9, pp 273-5.

Travers, T. (1998) 'The day of the watchdog', *Public Finance*, 16-22 October, pp 12-14.

Tunstill, J., Aldgate, J., Wilson, M. and Sutton, P. (1996) 'Crossing the organisational divide: family support services', *Health and Social Care in the Community*, vol 4, no 1, pp 41-9.

Twinn, S. (1993) 'Principles in practice: a re-affirmation', *Health Visitor*, vol 66, no 9, pp 319-21.

Utting, W. (1991) *Children in the public care: A review of residential child care*, London: HMSO.

van Dijk T.A. (1997) *Discourse as structure and process*, London: Sage Publications.

Walby, S. and Greenwell, J. (1994) *Medicine and nursing: Professions in a changing health service*, London: Sage Publications.

Walsh, K. (1995) *Public services and market mechanisms: Competition, contracting and the new public management*, Basingstoke: Macmillan.

Warner, U. (1993) 'Improving input to case conferences', *Nursing Standard*, vol 7, no 22, p 33.

Watton, M. (1993) 'Regulation in child protection – policy failure?', *British Journal of Social Work*, vol 23, pp 139-56.

Webb, A. (1991) 'Co-ordination: a problem in public sector management', *Policy &Politics*, vol 19, no 4, pp 229-41.

Weber, M. (1978) *Economy and society: An outline of interpretive sociology*, Berkley, CA: University of California Press.

Webster, C. (1998) 'The BMA and the NHS', *British Medical Journal*, vol 317, pp 45-7.

Weir, S. and Hall, W. (1994) *Ego trip: Extra governmental organisations in the UK and their accountability*, Colchester: University of Essex and Charter 88 Trust.

Wensley, A. (1998) 'The value of story telling', *Knowledge and Process Management*, vol 5, no 1, pp 1-20.

West, M. and Field, R. (1995) 'Teamwork in primary care, 1: Perspectives from organisational psychology', *Journal of Interprofessional Care*, vol 9, no 2, pp 117-22.

Whittington, C. (1983) 'Social work in the welfare network', *British Journal of Social Work*, vol 13, no 3, pp 265-86.

Wiles, R. and Robison, J. (1994) 'Teamwork in primary care: the views and experiences of nurses, midwives and health visitors', *Journal of Advanced Nursing*, vol 18, pp 1202-11.

Wilkes, S. and Wright, M. (1987) 'Conclusion: comparing government–industry relations: states, sectors and networks', in S. Wilkes and M. Wright (eds) *Comparing government–industry relations: Western Europe, the United States and Japan*, Oxford: Clarendon Press.

Willcocks, A. (1967) *The creation of a national health service*, London: Routledge and Kegan Paul.

Wistow, G. (1982) 'Collaboration between health and local authorities: why is it necessary?', *Journal of Social Policy and Administration*, vol 16, no 1, pp 44-62.

Wistow, G. (1992) 'The health service policy community: professionals pre-eminent or under challenge?', in D. Marsh and R.A.W. Rhodes (eds) *Policy networks in British government*, Oxford: Oxford University Press.

Wistow, G., Hardy, B. and Leedham, I. (1993) 'Planning blight', *Health Service Journal*, 18 February, pp 22-4.

Witz, A. (1992) *Professions and patriarchy*, London: Routledge.

WOC (Welsh Office Circular) (1995) *Protecting children from abuse: The role of the education service* [WOC 52/95], Welsh Office.

World Development Report (1997) *The state in a changing world*, Oxford: World Bank and Oxford University Press.

Wright, V. (1994) 'Reshaping the state: implications for public administration', *West European Politics*, vol 17, pp 102-34.

Index